Book index

I0490147

Introduction to the book

Health benefits of pomegranate

Many studies have shown the benefits of pomegranate, especially its role in maintaining the integrity of the heart and arteries, so we will introduce you to its most prominent benefits in detail in this book

Pomegranate is a fruit originating from Persia, and it has been used since ancient times for various purposes due to the important nutrients it contains that have earned it many important benefits for health. Let us learn about the most important benefits of pomegranate as follows

benefits of pomegranate
Pomegranate is one of the most rich fruits in vitamins, minerals and antioxidants, and for this reason, eating it or drinking its natural juice offers many benefits, the most prominent of which are

1. Promote oral and dental health

Pomegranate is good for oral and dental health, as its use has been shown to contribute to reducing the risk of gingivitis.

Also, the use of a mouthwash that contains pomegranate daily for four weeks reduces the causes of oral diseases, and reduces the level of plaque accumulation on the teeth, due to the antioxidants present in pomegranate that contribute to preventing the accumulation of bacteria in the mouth.

2. Good for heart health

Pomegranate contributes to lowering high cholesterol and preventing the oxidation of harmful cholesterol, thus protecting against vascular occlusion, heart disease, and atherosclerosis.

3. Contribute to the prevention of cancer

Pomegranate is rich in antioxidants that contribute to strengthening the immune system and reducing cancer, and there are many existing studies on the benefits of pomegranate in fighting prostate cancer

4. Contribute to the prevention of anemia
The presence of high levels of iron in pomegranate made it a contributor to the prevention of anemia resulting from iron deficiency, in addition to the ability of iron to:

Helping relieve cases of arthritis.
Help treat eye infections.
Contribute to the prevention of osteoporosis.
5. Contribute to enhancing skin glow
Despite the many benefits of pomegranate in the medical field, it has also proven its effective role in the cosmetic field, as it contributes to slowing down aging, thanks to the unique components of antioxidants that work to protect the skin and cells from aging
All this and more we will get to know in this book

Pomegranate health benefits

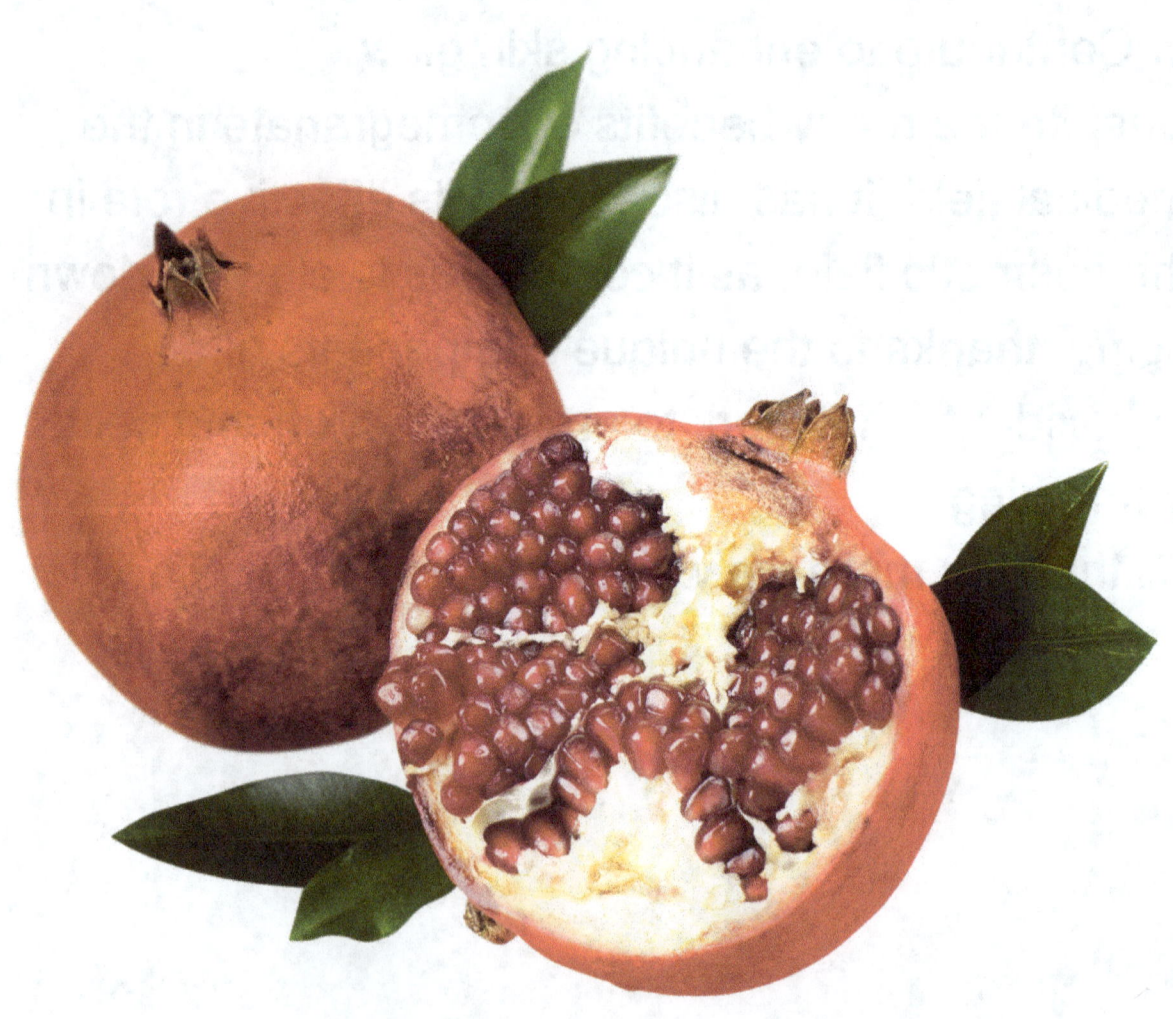

Pomegranate health benefits

Many studies have shown the benefits of pomegranate, especially its role in maintaining the integrity of the heart and arteries, so we will introduce you to its most prominent benefits in .detail in this book

Pomegranate health benefits
Pomegranate is a fruit originating from Persia, and it has been used since ancient times for various purposes due to the important nutrients it contains that have earned it many important benefits for health. Let us learn about the most prominent benefits of pomegranate as follows

benefits of pomegranate

Pomegranate is one of the most fruits rich in vitamins, minerals and antioxidants, so eating it or drinking its natural juice offers many benefits, the most prominent of which are:

1. Promote oral and dental health

Pomegranate is good for oral and dental health, as its use has been shown to reduce the risk of gingivitis.

The use of a mouthwash that contains pomegranate daily for four weeks reduces the causes of oral diseases, and reduces the level of plaque accumulation on the teeth, and the reason for this is due to the antioxidants present in pomegranate that contribute to preventing the accumulation of bacteria in the mouth.

2. Good for heart health

Pomegranate contributes to lowering high cholesterol and preventing the oxidation of harmful cholesterol, thus protecting against vascular blockage, heart disease, and atherosclerosis

3. Contribute to the prevention of cancer

Pomegranate is rich in antioxidants that contribute to strengthening the immune system and reducing cancer, and there are many studies based on the benefits of pomegranate in fighting prostate cancer.

4. Contribute to the prevention of anemia

The presence of high levels of iron in pomegranate made it a contributor to the prevention of anemia caused by iron deficiency, in addition to the ability of iron to:

Help relieve cases of arthritis.
Help treat eye infections.
Contribute to the prevention of osteoporosis.

5. Contribute to enhancing the freshness of the skin

Despite the many benefits of pomegranate in the medical field, it has also proven its effective role in the cosmetic field, as it contributes to slowing down aging, thanks to the unique antioxidant components that protect the skin and cells from aging

pomegranate juice benefits

The benefits of pomegranate juice include the following:

Strengthens the digestive system.

Contributes to the fight against diabetes.

It treats infections.

Contributes to protecting the heart from diseases.

Strengthens memory.

Improves fertility and sexual performance.

pomegranate pulp benefits

Among the most important benefits of eating pomegranate pulp are the following:

Reducing the risk of cardiovascular disease, heart attack and stroke, and lowering cholesterol and high pressure.

Reducing the risk of menopause-related diseases, such as osteoporosis, because the pomegranate pulp contains a substance similar to the effect of estrogen in the body.

Slowing the growth of cancer cells, thus reducing the risk of developing cancer, especially prostate cancer, breast cancer, and lymphoma.

Relieve diarrhea symptoms and strengthen immunity

Helping lose weight.

Prevention of cell damage and arthritis, as pomegranate has been shown to contain an enzyme that reduces or slows cartilage damage.

Help prevent diabetes.

Maintaining the skin, the pomegranate has a role in enhancing the absorption of vitamin D by enhancing the ability of skin cells to absorb it.

Benefits of pomegranate peel

The benefits of pomegranate can be obtained through the use of pomegranate peel, which has many benefits as follows:

1. Direct use of peels

The pomegranate peel is used directly for external treatment, as it works on the following:

Stop external bleeding.

Prevention of infections and various infections

2. Boiled pomegranate peels

In this method, dried pomegranate peels are boiled with water, and then the water is drunk after filtering to get many benefits, which include the following:

Protection from digestive problems and stomach disorders.

Prevention of colon problems.

Promote kidney and liver health.

Contribute to the elimination of parasites.

Pomegranate oil benefits

The benefits of pomegranate can also be obtained from its oil, which some people do not realize the importance of eating, as it can help in the following:

Nourishing the skin and giving it freshness and beauty.

Lowering cholesterol and blood sugar levels.

Lowering the level of blood pressure.

Fighting and destroying cancer

Pomegranate uses in ancient medicine

After you have learned about the most prominent benefits of pomegranate, here are its most prominent uses in ancient medicine:

Treating stomach worms.

Contribute to the treatment of sore throat.

Dysentery treatment.

Help treat sore eyes.

Contribute to wound healing.

Regulating the work of the digestive system.

Relieve nausea and headache.

Nutrients in pomegranate

The benefits of pomegranate stem from its richness in many nutrients, and here are the most prominent of them:

Antioxidants

Pomegranate contains flavonoid-type antioxidants and polyphenols, which together work as a very effective disease-fighting and anti-disease agent

fiber

The proportion of fiber in 100 grams of pomegranate is about 4 grams, which gives the body 12% of the recommended amount per day, and this made the pomegranate a good helper in preventing constipation, many chronic diseases, and cancers. Water and carbohydrates

A pomegranate contains 80% of its weight in water and 12% in carbohydrates, and a medium-sized pomegranate gives approximately 51 calories, and thus a pomegranate can be used in weight loss recipes.

vitamin C

Pomegranate is a good source of vitamin C, as 100 grams of pomegranate provides about 17% of our daily need for vitamin C, which is very important for strengthening immunity, and pomegranate contains many other vitamins such as: Vitamin K, which is necessary for blood clotting.

Nutrients

Pomegranate contains: iron, calcium, copper, manganese, and potassium, which are important for heart health

Pomegranate side effects

Pomegranate is a complex of therapeutic and health benefits necessary to protect our bodies and fortify them against many diseases. Its harm lies in the following:

Pomegranate impedes the absorption of some medications or affects their effect, so you should consult your doctor or pharmacist about this.

Pomegranate raises the level of sugar in the blood, and specialists have warned against eating large quantities of it because it contains a high percentage of sugar, especially for diabetics and those who suffer from a high level of fats in the blood

Buying and saving pomegranate
To obtain the benefits of pomegranate, it is preferable to buy dark-colored, large and heavy pomegranates for their size.

Pomegranate can be kept at normal room temperature, and in a dark place away from sunlight for about 5-8 days, or it can be kept in the refrigerator for about two to three weeks without removing the peel.

However, it is preferable to extract the grains from the fruit and store them in an airtight plastic container, where they can be kept for two weeks in the refrigerator, and in the freezer or freezer for more than ten months

Study on the benefits and health properties of pomegranate

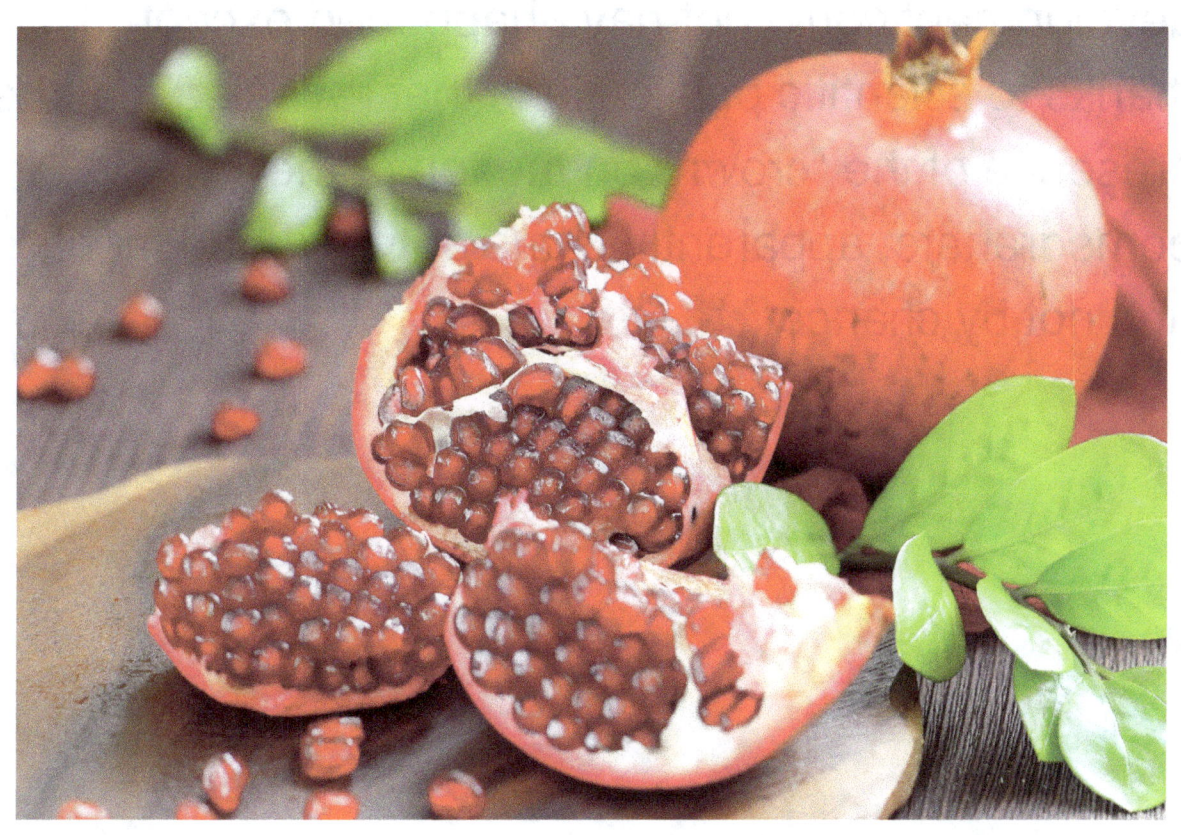

Study on the benefits and health properties of pomegranate

Laboratory studies have proven that many components of pomegranate have the ability to .reduce the spread of cancerous cells

Study on the benefits and health properties of pomegranate

The pomegranate fruit, even a short time ago, was very oppressed in our shopping basket. But recent years have witnessed a noticeable rise in per capita consumption of pomegranate. Why? Because all this development could not have happened except thanks to scientific publications that revealed that the presence of the "crown" on the top of the pomegranate, apparently came on merit and merit, and not by chance

Fruits are very important food in our diet. The fact is that we must increase our consumption of fruits, as they – in addition to vegetables – are our first and most important source of dietary fiber and "phytochemicals" (phytochemicals – plant chemicals that play a role in plants, such as pigments or colors, and have a significant contribution to human health).

If we adhere to the minimum recommendations that indicate that we should consume at least 5 servings of fruits and vegetables per day (noting that an increase in this area leads to what is better and does not harm), then our health will improve and our chances and risks of disease will decrease.

Fruits have many important health properties, many of which we are not aware of. Pomegranate is one of these fruits, and it has recently received a lot of scientific support, as it has been shown to be rich in chemical compounds (such as phytochemicals of the type polyphenols). Laboratory studies have shown that many components of pomegranate have the ability to reduce the spread of cancer cells

In a clinical research, during which a number of adults drank pomegranate juice and apple juice for 4 weeks, it was found that the group that drank pomegranate juice showed a significant improvement in antioxidant resistance. Also, the group of heart patients showed a significant improvement after drinking pomegranate juice for a period of 3 weeks, compared to the control group. As for the athletes, taking nutritional supplements containing pomegranate extracts improved their ability to recover in the post-workout phase, and to build up the necessary strength during the days following the training itself.

Pomegranate is richer in antioxidants than green tea, and is refreshing and delicious when added to salads, eaten on its own, or even added as juice to sauces

Calories in pomegranate and its most prominent benefits

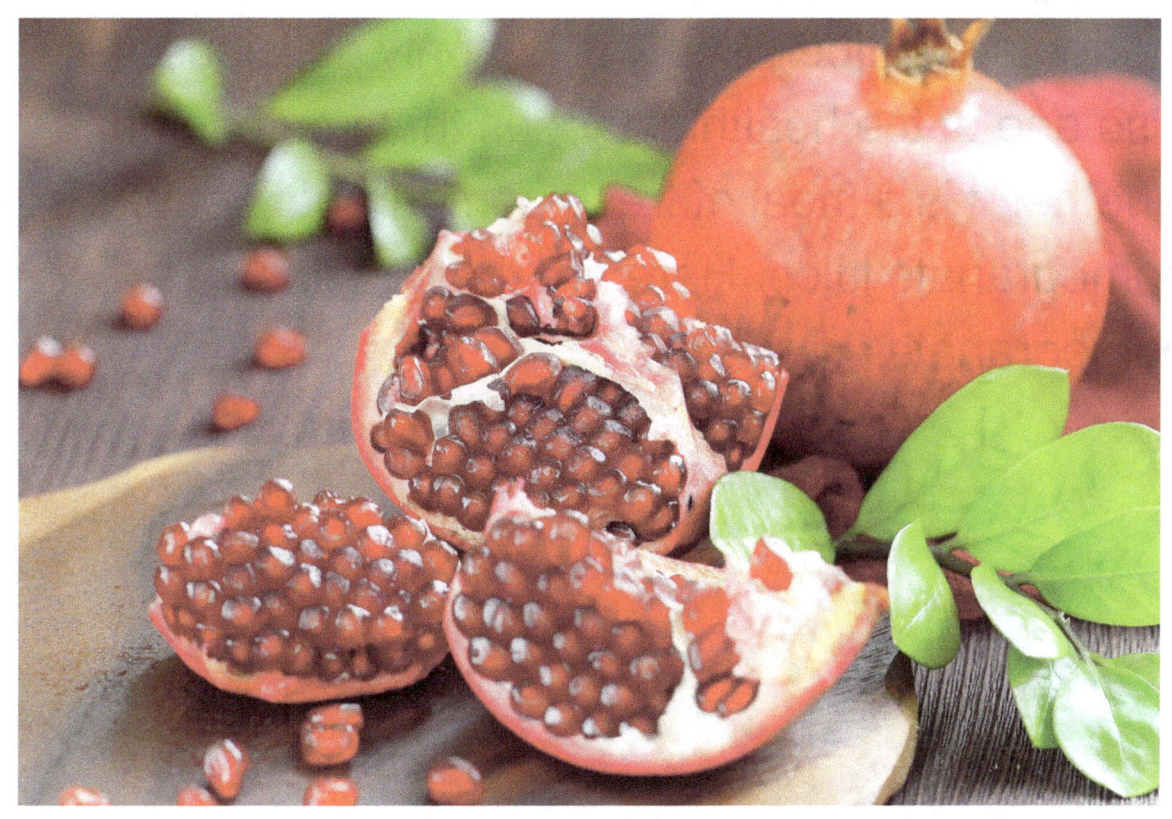

Calories in pomegranate and its most prominent benefits

Learn about the calories in pomegranate, its health benefits and some caveats when eating it in the following article.

Calories in pomegranate and its most prominent benefits
Pomegranate is one of the fruits that is very rich in nutrients and fiber, and it is not only delicious, but also one of the healthiest foods that you can eat, whether it is a meal of fresh pomegranate seeds or pomegranate juice. Here are the calories in pomegranate

Calories in pomegranate

Here are the calories in pomegranate and the nutritional value of one cup of fresh seeds as follows:

Contents

Nutritional value in pomegranate / cup

Calories in pomegranate

145 calories

water 136 gr

protein 2.9 grams

Total fat 2 grams

Carbohydrates 32.7 gr

7 grams of fiber

sugar 23.9 gr

Calcium 17.5 milligrams

Magnesium 21 milligrams

Potassium 413 milligrams

Vitamin C 17.5 milligrams

The health benefits of pomegranate

After knowing the calories in pomegranate, here are some of its health benefits:

1. It is rich in antioxidants

Pomegranate contains three times more antioxidants than other fruits. It also acquires its beautiful color from polyphenols, which are among the most powerful antioxidants that help protect cells from damage and prevent infections.

2. Prevents cancer

Recently found the effect of pomegranate juice on the prevention of prostate cancer.

3. Good for gut health

Pomegranate helps reduce inflammation in the intestines, it is very beneficial for patients with gastrointestinal and ulcerative colitis, and it also improves digestion.

4. Prevents Alzheimer's

The antioxidants in pomegranate help delay the progression of Alzheimer's disease and improve memory

5. Protects against arthritis

Flavonols in pomegranate prevent inflammation in the joints and reduce cartilage damage.

6. It is important for the health of the heart and arteries

Pomegranate juice improves blood flow and helps protect arteries from hardening and cholesterol buildup.

7. It increases immunity

The vitamins in pomegranate, such as: vitamin C and vitamin E, help boost immunity, and it has been found that pomegranate is antibacterial and common viruses and contributes to fighting infections.

8. It is rich in Vitamin C

A cup of pomegranate juice contains 40% of your daily requirement for vitamin C, which is important for iron absorption and wound healing, as well as for building healthy bones, muscles and cartilage

9. It lowers blood pressure

It was found that there is an ability of pomegranate juice to lower systolic and diastolic blood pressure, so it is important for people at risk of high blood pressure.

10. Regulates blood sugar

The amount of fiber present in pomegranate helps slow down the absorption of sugar, thus helping to prevent a rise in blood sugar after eating meals

Tips when eating pomegranate

Here are some tips to get the benefits of pomegranate and add the calories in pomegranate to your diet:

Always choose ripe, hard-skinned fruit. Because it tastes better and is easier to peel, and small scratches do not affect the quality of the fruit.

Just eat the seeds and discard the white part inside. Although safe to eat, it gives a bitter taste.

Store frozen pomegranate seeds in the freezer for up to 12 months and enjoy them the rest of the year.

Add pomegranate to green salads and mixed fruit salads.

Put some pomegranate seeds in your breakfast with oatmeal and yogurt for a more filling meal.

Use pomegranate as a garnish on dessert dishes.

Make a delicious smoothie with pomegranate seeds or add them to other cocktails.

Use pomegranate juice with a little sugar and spices to make a dip for grilled chicken and shrimp

Tips when eating pomegranate

Here are some tips to get the benefits of pomegranate and add the calories in pomegranate to your diet:

1- Always choose ripe, hard-skinned fruits; Because it tastes better and is easier to peel, and small scratches do not affect the quality of the fruit.

2- Eat the seeds only and get rid of the white part inside. Although it is safe to eat, it gives a bitter taste.

3- Store the pomegranate seeds by freezing in the freezer for up to 12 months and enjoy them the rest of the year.

4- Add pomegranate in green salads and mixed fruit salads.

5- Add some pomegranate seeds to your breakfast with oatmeal and yogurt for a richer meal.

6- Use pomegranate as a decoration on dessert dishes.

7- Make a delicious smoothie out of pomegranate seeds or add them to other types of cocktails

8- Use pomegranate juice with a little sugar and spices to make a dip for the chicken
grilled shrimp

Special precautions for eating pomegranate

Some special cautions and precautions when consuming pomegranate seeds or juice are as follows:

Some people may be allergic to pomegranate juice, and symptoms include itching, swelling, runny nose, and difficulty breathing.

Avoid eating dried pomegranate peel in large quantities by mouth, as it is unsafe and contains a lot of toxins.

Avoid any kind of pomegranate extract during pregnancy and lactation, and stick only to pomegranate juice, as it is safe.

You should be careful not to drink pomegranate juice for people with low blood pressure. Because it slightly lowers blood pressure.

Stop drinking or eating pomegranate for two weeks before any surgery. Because it affects blood pressure control during and after surgery

The many benefits of pomegranate peel for your health

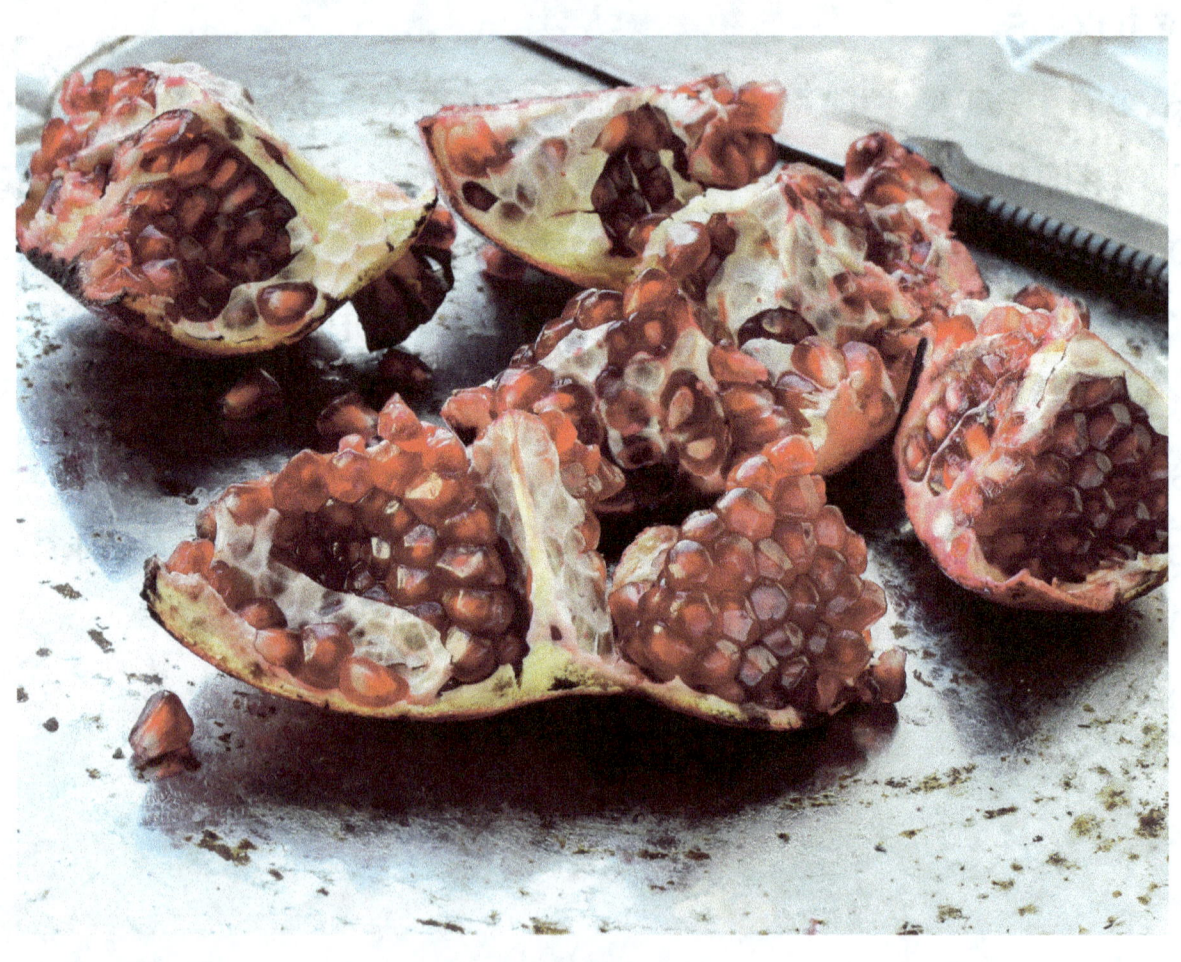

The many benefits of pomegranate peel for your health
Red pomegranate seeds are known as a source of antioxidants and fight many diseases, but what about the benefits of pomegranate peel

The pomegranate is considered one of the fruits with a delicious taste and many benefits for the health of the body. It has always been described in ancient medicine to treat many diseases, in addition to what modern medicine has proven to do with its role in fighting cancer, treating it and preventing many other health problems. What are the most important benefits of peel? pomegranate

Benefits of boiled pomegranate peel

It is possible to boil dried pomegranate peels and drink the water after filtering it to obtain many benefits that include:

Treating digestion problems and stomach disorders.
Control of colon problems.
Promote kidney and liver health.
An ideal drink to eliminate parasites.
Pomegranate peel powder or dried peels can be boiled with a herbal mixture containing: mint, ginger, cumin, and green tea with a small spoonful of honey, to get an immune-boosting and parasite-repelling drink.

Or it is possible to collect these ingredients in their dry form and grind them together, then add a spoonful of them to a cup of boiling water and drink it, and then add honey to it

The benefits of crushed pomegranate peel and how to use it

Crushed pomegranate peel can be used to treat several health problems by using several recipes:

To get rid of bad breath: Take a tablespoon of ground pomegranate peel to treat bad breath.

To lower blood pressure, reduce stress, and promote heart health: Drink a cup of decoction of crushed pomegranate peel daily.

To get rid of sore throat: eat a tablespoon of pomegranate peel powder or gargle with its water after boiling it.

Strengthening bones and enhancing their health: Eating boiled pomegranate peel with lemon juice and salt helps reduce bone density loss, thus preventing osteoporosis

Dry the pomegranate peel

When we talk about pomegranate peel, we mean here the complete inner and outer peel surrounding the seeds only without the inner yellow pulp with a bitter taste. We will talk to you here in particular about the benefits of pomegranate peel and how to use it:

How to dry pomegranate peels?

The process of drying pomegranate peels is usually done by applying the following:

Take a fresh pomegranate and cut it in half from the middle.

Cut them into four sections to make it easier to remove the red seeds and bitter pulp.

Take the outer rinds and cut them into smaller pieces to make the drying process easier.

Place it on a dry cloth and expose it to direct sunlight.

After it is completely dried, you can use it as is or grind it using a mortar.

Keep it in an airtight bag or in a special box

Benefits of pomegranate peel for the skin
Pomegranate peel has many benefits for skin, hair and beauty, which include:

Pomegranate peel powder is a natural moisturizer for the skin: it can be mixed with milk and applied to the face for ten minutes, then washed with cold water.

A natural skin exfoliator to remove dead cells: brown sugar can be mixed with pomegranate peel powder and olive oil and used to exfoliate the skin by massaging it and then washing it with lukewarm water.

Sun protection and reduced risk of skin cancer: Mix pomegranate peel powder with a group of essential oils and vitamin E, then apply it to your skin as a natural sunscreen.

Treating acne and fighting pimples: mix pomegranate peel powder with a little rose water and apply it on the face for 20 minutes

Fighting wrinkles and signs of aging: Use pomegranate peel powder with olive oil, avocado, or milk, apply it for a quarter of an hour on the face, and then wash it with lukewarm water.

Promotes healthy hair and strengthens it: thanks to its content of minerals and antioxidants, it also fights dandruff.

Benefits of pomegranate peel

It was found that pomegranate peels may help promote general health and treat some diseases when consumed, due to their content of:

Flavonoids.

Phenolic compounds.

Tannins.

A variety of minerals, such as: potassium, magnesium, sodium, calcium, phosphorus and complex sugars.

Here are the most important benefits of these pomegranate peels

1– Prevention of heart disease

Powerful antioxidants are present in the red pomegranate seeds as well as in their peels such as; Flavonoids and phenolic compounds.

Where it helps in combating infections and diseases of the heart and arteries, and the pomegranate peel is a source of potassium and magnesium, which are two very important elements for the functioning of the heart and arteries and the regulation and control of blood pressure.

In addition, eating boiled ground pomegranate peel contributes to reducing blood cholesterol levels and helps combat atherosclerosis

2- Promoting the health of the gastrointestinal tract
It was found that pomegranate peels have anti-inflammatory properties of the digestive system and intestines and facilitate the process of digestion, as they help stop bleeding in the intestines and enhance the functioning of its lining thanks to the content of some minerals such as potassium, magnesium and tannins, and thus they help in the prevention and treatment of diarrhea.

Pomegranate peel is also considered a repellent for parasites and worms that may be inside the intestines, and it contributes to promoting colon health and preventing hemorrhoids. Consult the specialist doctor and therapist before that

3- Treatment of sore throat

Pomegranate peel can contribute to soothing the symptoms of tonsillitis and throat, thanks to its anti-inflammatory properties and thanks to the powerful antioxidants it contains, such as; Flavonoids, and in this case it is used by boiling a group of dried pomegranate peels or their powder in water and then drinking the boil.

Or you can gargle with it, as this will help you reduce tonsil pain and sore throat as well in some cases

4- Promoting oral and dental health

Among the benefits of pomegranate peel is that it helps in treating a range of oral and dental problems by cleansing the mouth and balancing the bacteria environment in it, and among these problems that it works to combat:

Bad breath problem.

tooth decay.

Gingivitis.

mouth ulcers

In this case, it is applied by gargling twice a day with a mixture of one tablespoon of crushed dry pomegranate peel with a cup of water to eliminate bad breath, or rub the gums with powder to reduce swelling and to fight cavities

5- Promoting bone health

It was found that eating pomegranate peel powder can contribute to reducing the loss of bone density and preventing osteoporosis, especially in the post-forty and menopause stage, thanks to its content of calcium and phosphorus.

In addition, its anti-inflammatory properties contribute to promoting bone and joint health, as it is recommended to drink a mixture of pomegranate peel powder with lemon juice to obtain this benefit.

6- The benefits of pomegranate peel for slimming

It may sometimes be advised to try a decoction of pomegranate peel in the matter of weight loss and diets. Drinking a decoction of pomegranate peel with ginger or mint may:

Helps facilitate digestion and excretion.

Encourages metabolism and fat burning in the body.

Helps you feel full and reduce the amount of food you eat during the day.

We also advise you to drink this boiled one to two times per day to collect this benefit in such cases

7- The benefits of pomegranate peel for the stomach

Dried pomegranate peel, when consumed in boiled or powdered form, improves the health of the digestive system and stomach thanks to its content of antioxidants, anti-inflammatory and tannins. Pomegranate peel also works to treat stomach acidity problems, ulcers and infections, and relieve symptoms.

It is recommended to eat a mixture of dried pomegranate peel powder with milk and rock salt to treat digestion problems

Benefits of pomegranate peel for hair

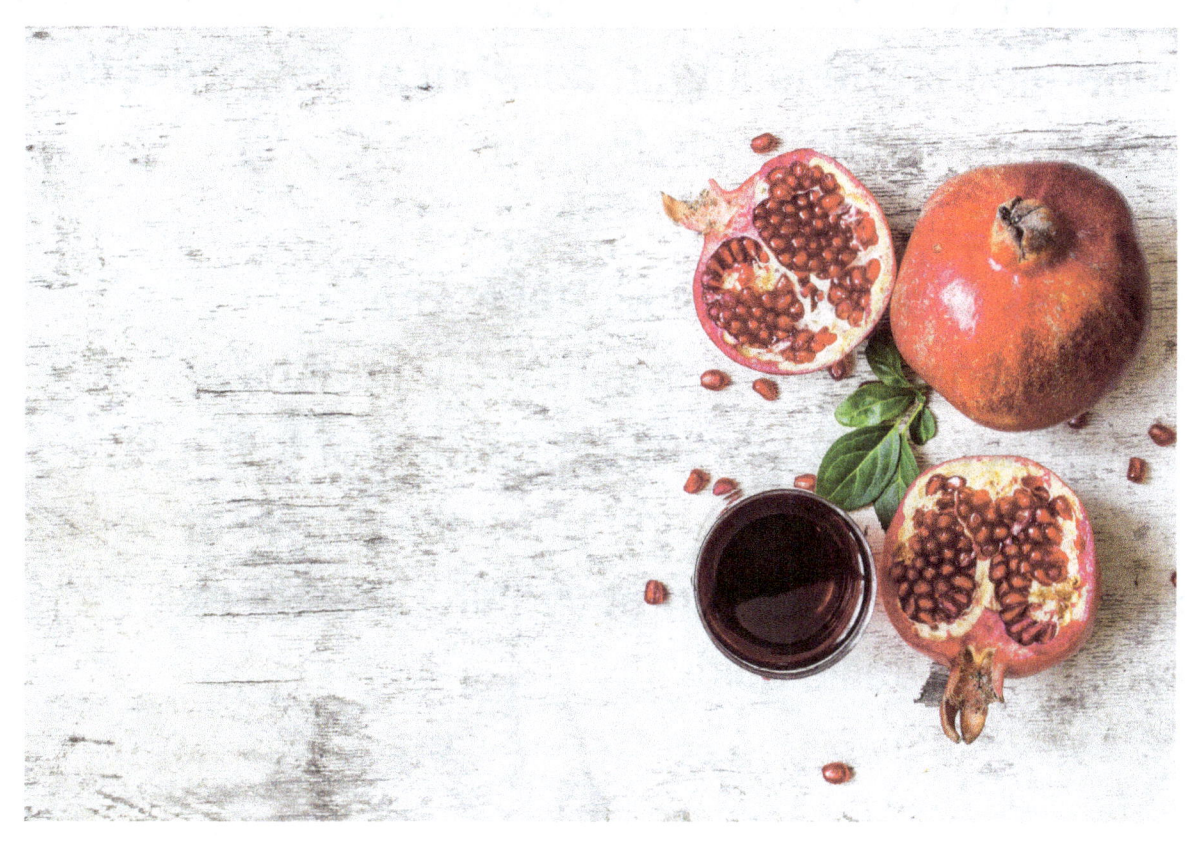

Benefits of pomegranate peel for hair

Pomegranate peel contains many vitamins and minerals necessary for hair, so what are the benefits of pomegranate peel for hair? How can it be used?

Benefits of pomegranate peel for hair
Perhaps you were one of the people who eat pomegranates and get rid of their peels thinking that they are useless, but they contain vitamins and minerals that benefit hair, so what are the benefits of pomegranate peels for hair?

Benefits of pomegranate peel for hair
Pomegranate peels contain many healthy components that increase the value of this fruit, such as: antioxidants and phenolic compounds such as: flavonoids, anthocyanins, catechins, tannin, and gallic acid

This group straightens the hair from its roots and ends.

Among the benefits of pomegranate peel for hair is that it reduces hair problems, as minerals and vitamins can help nourish the scalp and its roots, and among its other benefits, we mention the following:

Strengthening hair follicles.
Help reduce baldness problems.
Helping to increase the intensity of hair loss.
Preventing premature graying.
Addressing annoying dandruff problems by treating dry scalp.
Counting hair with vitamins is dedicated to hair growth.
And the idea of hair dyes to add red color.
Ways to use pomegranate peels for hair cognitive quadrants

Pomegranate peel mask

To get the benefits of pomegranate peel for hair here, follow these steps:

1 Cut the pomegranate into very small pieces and soak them in water until they are covered.

2 Bring to a boil over low heat until the liquid becomes very thick, then set aside to cool.

3 Put the mixture on the hair where you can use a spray bottle and massage the scalp with it, you can repeat this process twice a week to get the desired result.

4 Add a spoonful of yogurt to the decoction of pomegranate peel if your scalp is of the oily type, while if it is dry, you can add mashed avocado fruit to form a paste that can be spread on the scalp.

5 Leave the mixture on the hair for 20 minutes before washing it with shampoo as usual.

Pomegranate peel powder mask

You can use pomegranate peel as a base to get the benefits of pomegranate peel for hair through the following steps:

1 Mix three tablespoons of pomegranate peel base, three more tablespoons of pomegranate blossom base, three tablespoons of chamomile base, and a little lemon juice.

2 Heat the mixture well and leave it for a while until it becomes warm.

Apply to the hair before taking a shower for two 3 hours, then repeat this process twice a week

Pomegranate peel for dyed hair
Pomegranate peel helps maintain the color of red
hair by washing red-dyed hair with pomegranate
peel infusion.

Side effects of using pomegranate peel on hair
There is not enough scientific evidence to prove
the degree of safety of using pomegranate peel on
the scalp, so you should be careful and test a small
amount of the previously mentioned recipes on a
small part of the scalp to ensure that no unwanted
side effects appear before using it completely.
Other benefits of pomegranate peel for the body
In addition to the benefits of pomegranate peel for
hair, pomegranate peels may contain many
vitamins, minerals and antioxidants, through which
benefits can be obtained, including:
1. Promote a healthy body
Due to the abundance of antioxidants in
pomegranate peels, they can help lower
cholesterol levels, especially bad cholesterol,
protect the heart, and prevent harmful fats from
oxidizing in your body

It can also prevent bacteria, thus reducing inflammation and treating colon problems.

2. Detoxification of the body

The antioxidants present in pomegranate peel can help detoxify the internal organs in the body and keep the body systems functioning well.

3. Providing a large amount of vitamin C to the body

You can get a very good amount of vitamin C from pomegranate peel, which works to strengthen the body's immunity and quickly relieve wounds and scars.

Vitamin C also helps build body mass by forming essential proteins and repairing cartilage damage.

4. Maintaining dental health

Pomegranate peels are often used to keep teeth clean and healthy, as they reduce bad breath.
While pomegranate peels are included in toothpaste formulations

5. Help treat a sore throat

You can use pomegranate peel powder and warm water to relieve a sore throat by gargling with the mixture, and this mixture can give you quick relief from sore throat pain.

6. Help treat

The vitamins and minerals present in pomegranate peels can help alleviate skin problems, as they are an effective moisturizer for the skin, and protect it from harmful sunlight, especially ultraviolet.

It may also help remove burns in the skin, reduce signs of aging, such as: wrinkles and pigmentation, and keep your skin bright, glowing and supple

Benefits of pomegranate peel for the stomach and body

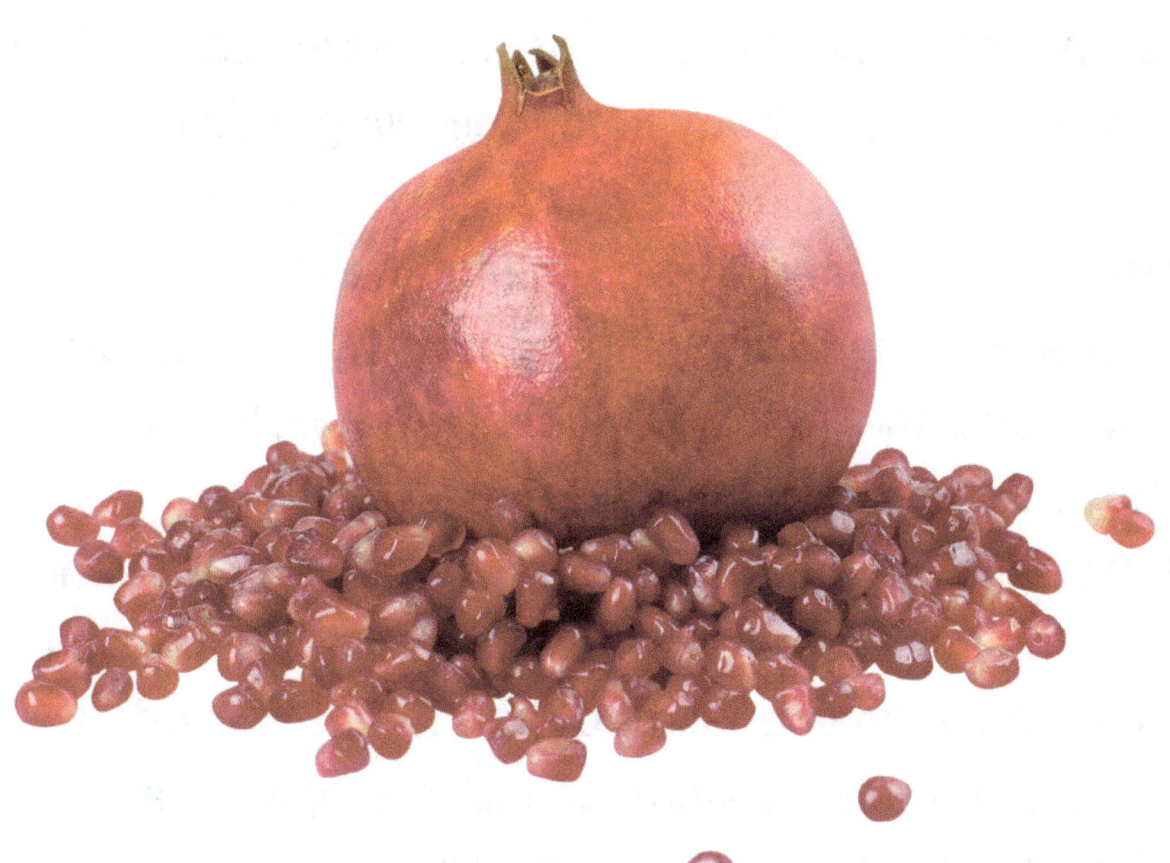

Benefits of pomegranate peel for the stomach and body
Pomegranate is characterized by its many benefits on the body, and it is one of the seasonal fruits that many await for its delicious taste. Learn about the benefits of pomegranate peel for the stomach in the following article.

Benefits of pomegranate peel for the stomach and body
Pomegranate has many benefits for the body. Let's learn about the benefits of pomegranate peel for the stomach and body in the following article:

Benefits of pomegranate peel for the stomach
There are many benefits offered by pomegranate peel, and the most prominent and well-known of these benefits are the following:
It helps in the process of calming the stomach and calming its various disorders, as pomegranate is a powerful antibacterial, and therefore it is used as a natural remedy for stomach disorders, such as: diarrhea, dysentery, and cholera

Drinking tea made from pomegranate leaves may help get rid of indigestion.

A 2005 study revealed that pomegranate extracts have stomach-benefiting properties due to their high concentration of antioxidants, and can be used to treat abdominal cramps and discomfort.

Health benefits of pomegranate peel

After we have mentioned the most important benefits of pomegranate peel for the stomach, we must now mention the most prominent and famous benefits for health in general, the most important of which are the following:

1. Works as a natural sunscreen

Pomegranate peels contain sunscreens that protect your skin from UV rays, which can cause skin cancer.

2. It acts as a natural facial exfoliator

Pomegranate peel can act as a natural facial exfoliator, as it removes white and blackheads and dead skin if it is added to facial exfoliating mixtures

3. Fights wrinkles and symptoms of aging

Pomegranate peel helps fight aging and wrinkles that make your skin look younger, it helps prevent the breakdown of collagen which maintains youthful and healthy skin.

4. Works as a natural moisturizer

The components of pomegranate peel are excellent for the skin, as it soothes the skin and protects it from toxins and environmental pollutants. The pomegranate peel also contains lactic acid, which helps retain moisture inside the body and keeps it healthy and soft.

5. Fights acne, pimples and rashes

Pomegranate peels are rich in antioxidants, and their use helps protect the skin from bacteria and other inflammatory causes, and fights acne, pimples and rashes.

6. Sore throat healer

After knowing the benefits of pomegranate peel for the stomach, that if you suffer from a sore throat, inflammation, or pain in the tonsils, you can gargle with boiled pomegranate peel powder to soothe your pain

7. Antibacterial and antiviral

In a study published in 2012, it was found that pomegranate peels contain a wide range of important and beneficial antioxidants for the body, and it was noted that they have a role in fighting various viruses and bacteria.

The study suggested the possibility of using pomegranate peels as a natural source to fight various bacteria, viruses and germs.

8. Reducing hair loss

Another benefit of pomegranate peel is that it works to reduce hair loss and fight scalp dandruff, as this is due to the properties and nutrients that pomegranate peel contains.

To obtain this benefit, it is possible to combine pomegranate peel powder with the hair oil that you use, then apply it to the roots of the hair and massage the scalp, and after about two hours, the hair must be washed with shampoo

Side effects of pomegranate peel
There are many benefits of pomegranate peel for
the health and aesthetics of the stomach, but there
are also some side effects and damages that may
result from its use and consumption, the most
prominent of which are the following:

Suffering from some allergic reactions.
flushing
itching
Runny nose.
breathing difficulties

Benefits of pomegranate peel for the vagina: do they exist?

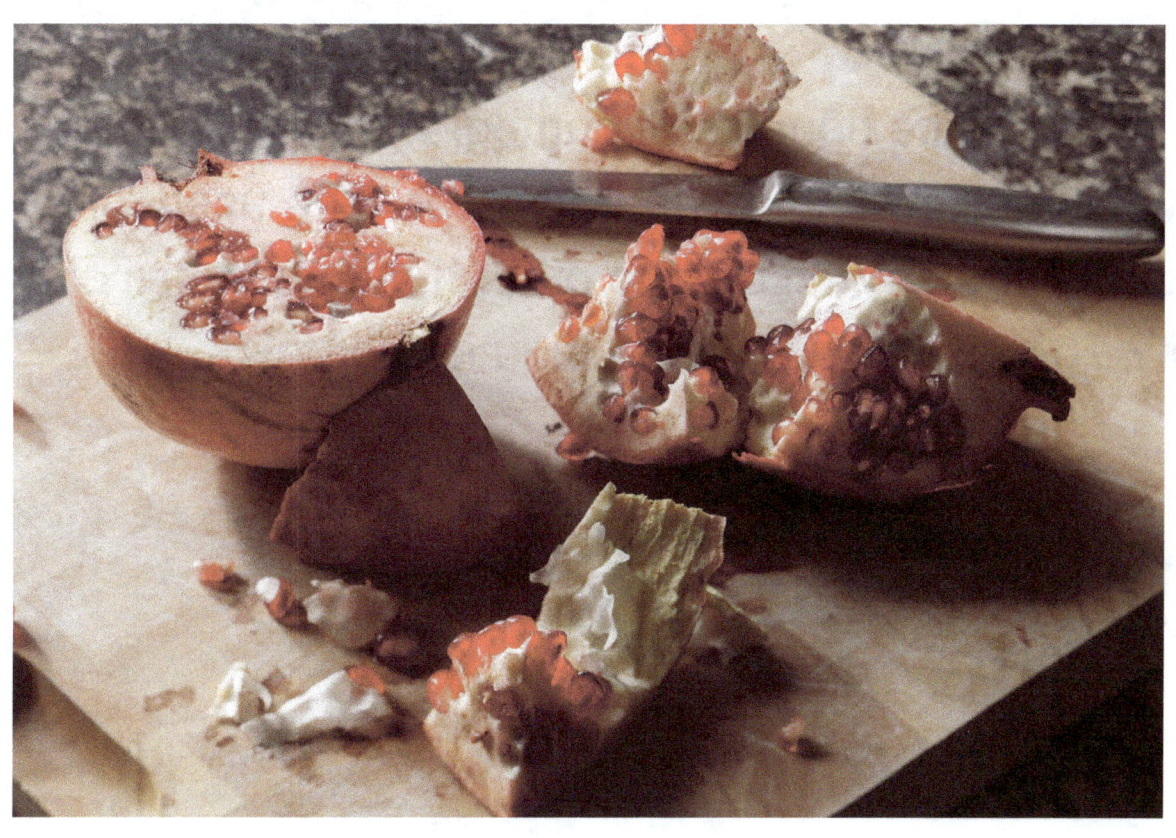

Benefits of pomegranate peel for the vagina: do they exist?

Pomegranate is one of the fruits that has many health benefits, but what are the benefits of pomegranate peel for the vagina? What are the benefits of eating pomegranate for the vagina? All this and more, we will learn about it in the following article.

Benefits of pomegranate peel for the vagina: do they exist?
What are the benefits of pomegranate peel for the vagina? How can pomegranate peel be used for the vagina? What are the other health benefits of it? The following is an explanation for this

What are the benefits of pomegranate peel for the vagina?

The expected benefits of pomegranate peel for the vagina will be explained in the following:

A study showed that pomegranate peel or its extracts contribute to strengthening the muscles of the pelvic floor of women, which increases their sexual pleasure.

Pomegranate extracts and their peels contribute to the treatment of vaginal atrophy, especially in menopause, which causes pain during intercourse and painful urinary symptoms, according to a study. Eating pomegranate contributes to maintaining the health of the vagina in general, and this can be reflected in pomegranate peels as well, so we will explain in the following points the expected benefits of pomegranate on the vagina:

Pomegranate is rich in phytoestrogens.

It fights vaginal infections by preventing the growth of microorganisms because it contains antibiotics.

Reduces unwanted vaginal secretions for its role in improving its pH and balance

How can pomegranate peel be used?
The benefits of pomegranate peel for the vagina
are many and varied, and to benefit from it, one of
the following recipes must be used:

Pomegranate peel powder tea
Pomegranate peel powder tea can be prepared at
home by using the following ingredients and
following the next steps:

1- Separate the peels from the pomegranate.
2- Place the peels in a place exposed to direct
sunlight for 2-3 days or until they are completely
dry.
3- Transfer the dry peels to a food processor and
start grinding them until they turn into a powder.
4- Store the powder in an airtight container
5- Soak a quantity of pomegranate peel powder in
boiling water to enjoy pomegranate peel tea

Pomegranate peel lotion

Pomegranate peel lotion contributes to narrowing the vagina and cleansing the area. The lotion is prepared through the following ingredients and steps:

1- Wash the pomegranate peels, then place them in a dry place exposed to sunlight until they are completely dry.

2- Crush the dried peels using a food processor and store them in a bowl.

3- Put 1 liter of water in a pot and then put it on the stove until it boils and finally take it away so that the water becomes just hot.

4- Dissolve enough powder in hot water. Use the lotion once a month

5- During showering and on the outside area Vagina only

What are the other health benefits of pomegranate peel?

Here are a number of other health benefits of pomegranate peel:

1- It helps treat some skin problems because it contains antioxidants and polyphenols, and it also reduces hyperpigmentation that results in dark spots.

2- It reduces the chances of developing chronic diseases when taken as a dietary supplement, as it improves heart health and controls blood sugar levels.

3- It may prevent age-related hearing loss, as it is rich in antioxidants.

4- It fights Alzheimer's disease and improves brain function

5- Resists cancerous diseases and limits the extent of their growth and spread to contain scales Large amounts of Punicalagin

What are the side effects or harms of using pomegranate peel?

Here are a number of possible side effects and harms of pomegranate peel when used:

Allergic reactions that appear in the form of a rash and itching when used externally.

Swelling, runny nose, and difficulty breathing caused by allergies after eating pomegranate extracts or peels.

Taking pomegranate or its extracts by mouth, in large amounts, may not be safe

Pomegranate peel damage and benefits: what are they?

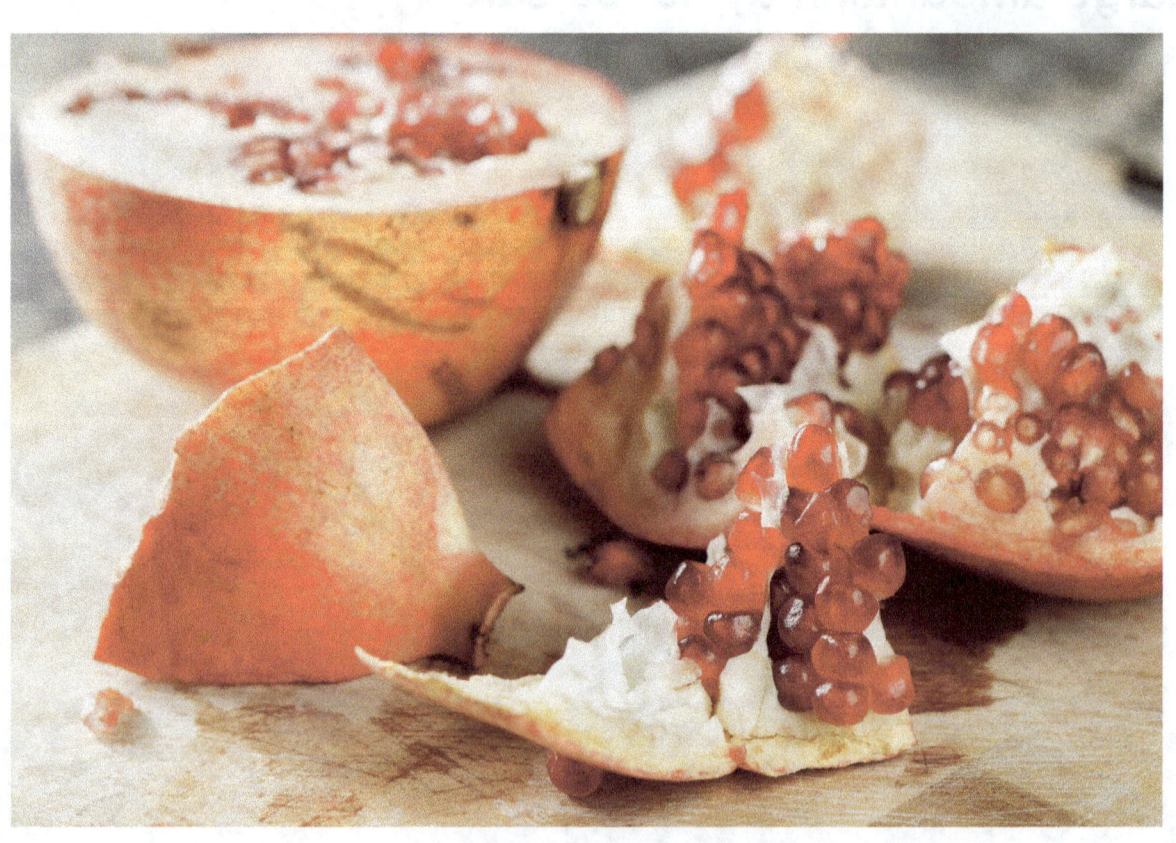

What are the side effects or harms of using pomegranate peel?

Here are a number of possible side effects and harms of pomegranate peel when used:

Allergic reactions that appear in the form of a rash and itching when used externally.

Swelling, runny nose, and difficulty breathing caused by allergies after eating pomegranate extracts or peels.

Taking pomegranate or its extracts by mouth, in large amounts, may not be safe

Pomegranate peel damage

Some people may be affected more than others by the effects of pomegranate peel, including:

Allergy sufferers suffer from pomegranate peel damage more than others. Because their immune system may respond to the pomegranate peel by triggering itching, swelling, blockage, and difficulty breathing.

Pomegranate peel affects the hormonal factor, as it increases the secretion of some hormones, which may later lead to serious complications.

Eating pomegranate peel powder without consulting a specialist can affect blood pressure and blood cholesterol.

Pomegranate peel affects the pH scale of the vaginal area when used, and the treatment of this problem may take longer than might be expected, and this is one of the disadvantages

Benefits of pomegranate peel

After identifying the damages of pomegranate peel, the many benefits of peel must be mentioned as follows:

There is pomegranate peel extract and vitamin C, which has been proven to be a successful treatment because its extract contains an effective substance to eliminate types of bacteria that are resistant to antibiotics.

It fights local infections caused by methicillin-resistant Staphylococcus aureus (MRSA).

It contains antioxidants that make it popular along with green tea and blueberries.

It is used to eliminate tapeworms, worms in general, and intestinal parasites that attack the human body.

Pomegranate peel is used to eliminate problems related to the digestive system along with many other natural ingredients.

There is some scientific evidence that rubbing the gums with pomegranate peel extract may improve gum disease

What research came about pomegranate peel

There is enough research to suggest that it is likely to be effective in lowering blood pressure, and some research shows that drinking pomegranate juice does not improve symptoms or breathing in people with lung disease.

Some research also shows that eating pomegranate does not lower cholesterol levels in people with high cholesterol.
Here's more about what the research came up with:

Atherosclerosis: Research shows that pomegranate juice can help protect the carotid arteries in the neck and reduce the accumulation of fat in them.

Physical performance: Early research shows that taking pomegranate extract might improve athletic performance.

Heart disease: Some research shows that pomegranate juice may improve blood flow to the heart, but there is not enough information about its relationship to heart disease and its symptoms

Teeth: Early research shows that using a mouthwash with pomegranate extract reduces plaque on the teeth.

Diabetes: Research shows that pomegranate syrup may help control blood sugar levels in people with diabetes.

Menopausal symptoms: Research shows that pomegranate seed oil extract improves sleep in some women with menopausal symptoms.

Muscle strength: Research shows that pomegranate extract can improve muscle strength after exercise.

Excess weight: Some research shows the benefit of some pomegranate products on overweight people, but there is an urgent need for more research in this regard.

Thrush: Applying a gel containing pomegranate extract to the gums may improve symptoms in people with thrush.

Rheumatoid arthritis: Little research shows that taking pomegranate extract can improve symptoms of rheumatoid arthritis.

Trichomoniasis: Some research has shown that eating pomegranate extract is related to relieving symptoms of Trichomoniasis in women

The benefits of eating pomegranate many and very important

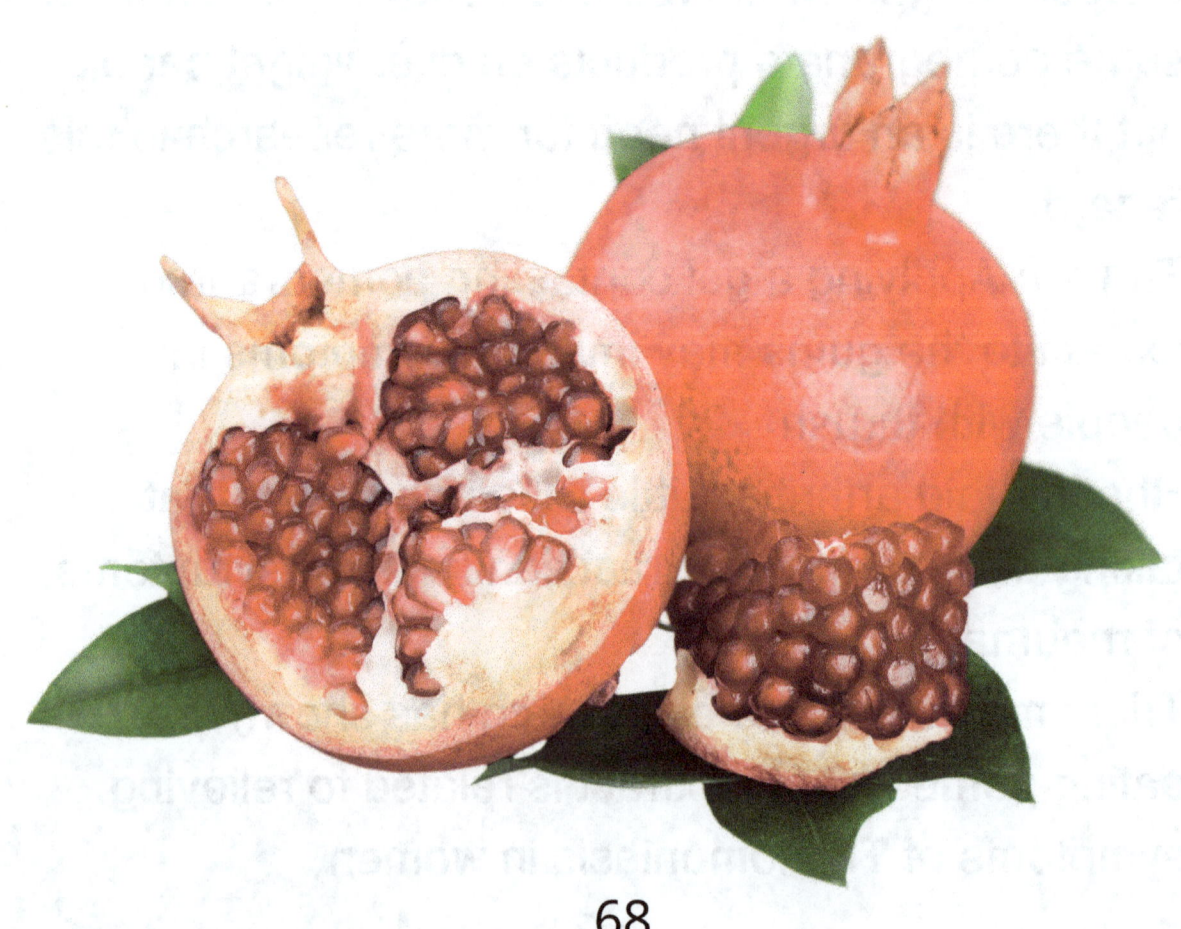

The benefits of eating pomegranate: many and very important

What are the benefits of eating pomegranate? How can eating pomegranate improve your health? Is it possible to eat pomegranate to return to you .damage? Details in the following article

The benefits of eating pomegranate: many and very important
Pomegranate is a delicious fruit scientifically known as Punica granatum. Pomegranate is characterized by its exceptional content of antioxidants in particular, in addition to many nutrients important for health, which make pomegranate a natural fruit that is nutritious and healthy. So what are the benefits of eating pomegranate? The answer awaits you in the following lines

Benefits of eating pomegranate

The benefits of eating pomegranates are not different from the benefits of natural pomegranate juice. Here is a list of the most important potential benefits of eating delicious pomegranate seeds:

1. Resistance to some types of cancer

Pomegranate contains very high amounts of antioxidants, in proportions that exceed some common foods and drinks rich in antioxidants, such as green tea. Antioxidants play an important role in resisting the state of oxidative stress and the free radicals that cause it, which can stimulate the emergence of cancer.

Therefore, thanks to the antioxidant content of pomegranates and many other important nutrients, eating pomegranates regularly can help:

Resisting the spread of prostate cancer cells, and accelerating their death.

Preventing certain types of cancers or resisting the spread of their cells after their origin, such as: breast cancer, colon cancer, lung cancer, and skin cancer

2. Reducing anemia

Pomegranate contains good proportions of iron, which plays an important role in promoting the production and pumping of blood, so eating pomegranate or drinking its natural juice regularly can help relieve anemia and many of the symptoms that may accompany it, such as:

Tired.

Loss or impairment of the sense of hearing.

general weakness.

Vertigo.

3. Strengthening your bones and joints and making them less susceptible to disease

Pomegranate pulp contains substances that may help support bone and joint health and resist some diseases that may affect them, such as the following:

Various antioxidants and natural anti-inflammatory substances, and these may help reduce inflammation and keep it under control, including infections that may play a role in the emergence of bone and joint diseases

Substances that may inhibit the production of enzymes whose activity can cause the breakdown of some connective tissue in the body. Therefore, one of the benefits of eating pomegranate is that it may help resist or slow down the pace of damage and degeneration that may affect cartilage, which may help keep the condition of osteoarthritis patients under control or delay the onset of the disease among candidates for infection, in addition to relieving the severity of symptoms of some other bone and joint diseases, Such as: rheumatoid arthritis.

4. Resistance to cardiovascular disease
Eating pomegranates for your circulatory system in particular may bring many benefits, such as:

Reducing high blood pressure, thanks to the high pomegranate content of some natural compounds that are believed to reduce pressure, such as: antioxidants

Substances that may inhibit the production of enzymes whose activity can cause the breakdown of some connective tissue in the body. Therefore, one of the benefits of eating pomegranate is that it may help resist or slow down the pace of damage and degeneration that may affect cartilage, which may help keep the condition of osteoarthritis patients under control or delay the onset of the disease among candidates for infection, in addition to relieving the severity of symptoms of some other bone and joint diseases, Such as: rheumatoid arthritis.

4. Resistance to cardiovascular disease
Eating pomegranates for your circulatory system in particular may bring many benefits, such as:

Reducing high blood pressure, thanks to the high pomegranate content of some natural compounds that are believed to reduce pressure, such as: antioxidants

Pomegranate: improves health and nourishes the skin

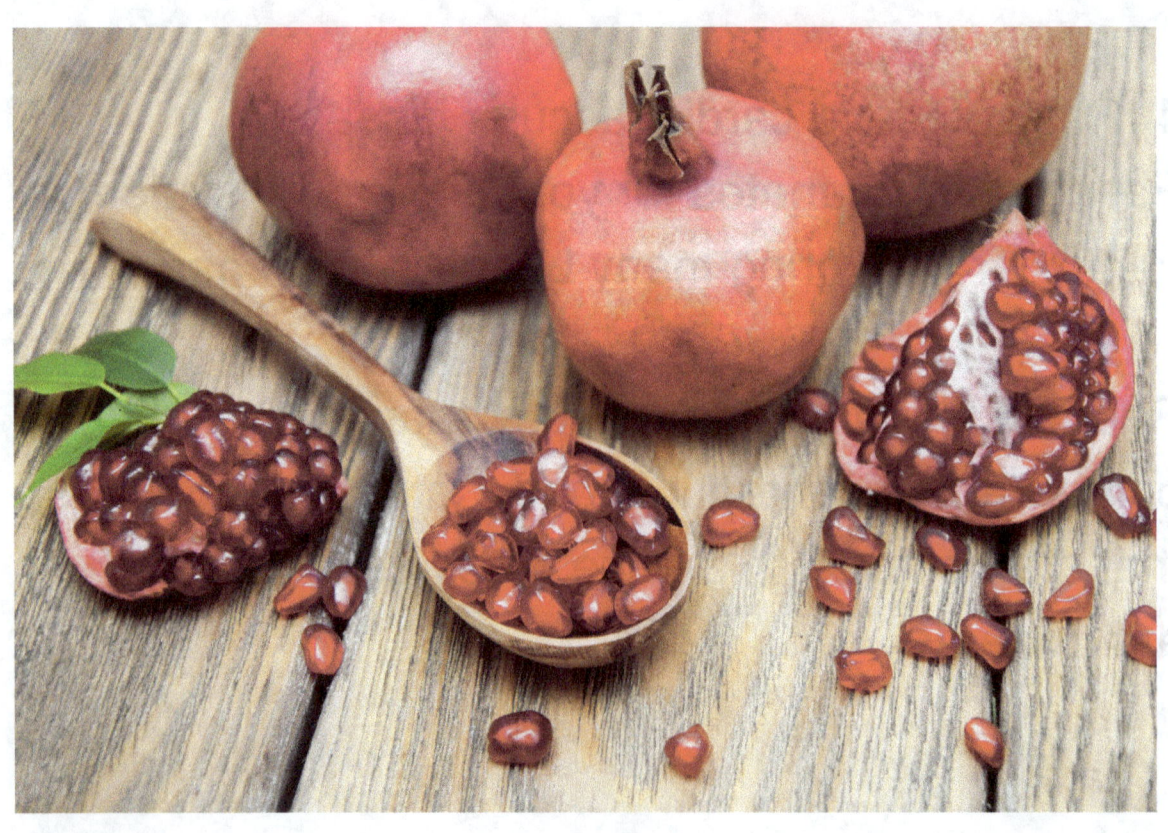

Pomegranate: improves health and nourishes the skin

Some may overlook the importance of eating pomegranate fruit, which is rich in oil that may help nourish your skin and give it freshness and beauty. It is also known for its ability to reduce cholesterol and blood sugar levels, in addition to lowering blood pressure. It is also known to combat and destroy cancer.

Pomegranate: improves health and nourishes the skin

It is a healthy fall fruit, rich in vitamins and minerals, and its fruits are concentrated in its original homeland, Iran, but its cultivation has spread in many warm Arab countries, and in the areas bordering the Mediterranean Sea. This pomegranate tree is considered by some to be a symbol of abundance and blessing as well as fertility and beauty, but it is used in the treatment of many health problems

There has been a lot of talk about the benefits of pomegranate and its multiple uses. The pomegranate fruit is included in the preparation of types of alcoholic cocktail juices, as well as the red granules mixed with some types of foods, and in the work of salads and baking. Also, the pomegranate has been known since ancient times for its role in making dyes for fabrics and leather, decorating and embellishing symbols and coins, Its extracted components are also included in the preparation of cosmetics and the treatment of some diseases.

One of the scientific studies conducted recently and on a large scale, demonstrating the importance of using pomegranate fruit oil extract in treating some health problems, which has been known since ancient times for its use in folk medicine in the Middle East, India and the Mediterranean. It is a unique oil and an important tool in treating a variety of diseases, including breast cancer treatment, cardiovascular diseases and strengthening the heart muscle as well

Studies have also shown the effect of pomegranate oil in lowering high blood pressure and blood sugar levels, as well as lowering the level of triglycerides and cholesterol in the blood.

The reason why pomegranate seed oil has effective capabilities in treating diseases is due to the fact that it contains important fatty acids, but its components are rich in additional effective compounds, among these compounds are the following:

Important fatty acids, the most important of which is conjugated linoleic acid - CLA, which is one of the important antioxidants, which was recently discovered. .
Polyphenols, a biologically active compound extracted from green plants with antioxidant qualities, destroy germs and viruses.
Vitamin E and gamma-tocopherol are among the most powerful antioxidant chemical compounds.
Pomegranate oil contains plant hormones

Pomegranate is a useful weapon for treatment
In addition to the therapeutic effect of pomegranate oil, the importance of pomegranate oil has recently been proven in the manufacture of cosmetic and beneficial products for skin care, especially since pomegranate seed oil is considered the richest compound with its benefits, which showed a clear and strong effect in caring for and nourishing the skin, as well as giving it a sense of vitality and a beautiful healthy appearance. The oil also has a role in slowing down the aging process of the skin and improving its appearance. However, it can treat facial skin and provide a useful solution to pigmentation problems.

The oil has natural estrogenic properties that contribute to skin renewal, filling in fine wrinkles, and helping to produce a lively and healthy appearance. The oil is characterized by containing the highest concentration of fatty acids used as antioxidants, which contribute to restoring skin cells and protecting it from pollution and treating wrinkles

Pure pomegranate oil is a rare and expensive commodity, and in order to prepare 15 cubic centimeters of pure pomegranate oil extract, 2.5 tons of pomegranate seeds are required, so the process of producing pomegranate oil is a complex and expensive process, and in order to extract it requires a precise separation process between the pulp of the pomegranate seed And between the shell of the seed, from which the oil is extracted. But in the end, after effort and time, you get a high quality oil that is useful for treatment.

It is reported that pomegranate seed oil contains 80% of antioxidants, which are associated with free radicals, and these antioxidants may disrupt and destroy the effect of free radicals. Free radicals are by-products of the metabolism of cells, and these radicals can damage and kill cells if the body fails to challenge them

So pomegranate is an important weapon for maintaining cardiovascular health, as studies have shown that daily consumption of pomegranate granules or drinking pomegranate juice may contribute to lowering "bad" LDL cholesterol levels in the blood, lowering blood pressure levels, improving blood flow to the heart, and preventing hardening of the arteries. . Thus, pomegranate can keep the heart safe from seizures and strokes, as well as cancer.

It is noteworthy that the fruits that contain the red pigments, and the purple group that contains anthocyanins, are powerful antioxidants that contribute to slowing the aging of the body and the brain, and these pigments possess antioxidant and anti-inflammatory properties and thus contribute along with the additional protective components in the pomegranate. However, Chinese medicine considers the red pigment in the pomegranate fruit to be a powerful blood tonic and beneficial for those suffering from anemia

Home recipes to clean the face

As we mentioned earlier, the benefits and uses of the pomegranate fruit and the oil extracted from it have multiplied, so you may resort to taking advantage of some homemade recipes that contain pomegranate oil, and these home recipes are useful for improving your skin.

Peeling for whitening and concealing blemishes

Peeling is intended for whitening spots concentrated on the face, and this method is useful for treating nicotine spots by using the hands. One tablespoon of water is mixed with a quarter of a spoonful of olive oil, the juice of one lemon, and a quarter of a spoonful of table salt and pomegranate juice. Where you paint the mixture on a clean face and massage while avoiding touching the eye area. This mixture is left on the face for an additional 10 minutes and then washed off with warm water. It is recommended to do this peeling once or twice a week

Exfoliating face and hands
This peeling helps to achieve a healthy and vibrant appearance, and is not suitable for delicate skin with capillaries. This peeling is done by applying a mixture of a tablespoon full of honey, two tablespoons of ground oatmeal, and a tablespoon of pomegranate juice. These ingredients are mixed well, then applied to the face, and the face and hands are massaged. Leave this mixture on the face for 10 minutes and then wash it well.

Pomegranate peeling for the face
This peeling is suitable for normal or oily skin, and it is used to remove dead cells and mainly clean the face. It is prepared by mixing a tablespoon full of honey with 3 tablespoons of ground almonds, putting a tablespoon of lemon juice, and a few pomegranate granules taken from half of the fruit. Then spread the paste on the face and rub it gently, and leave it on the face for 10 minutes and then wash it well to get clean skin

Benefits of pomegranate for men: fact or myth?

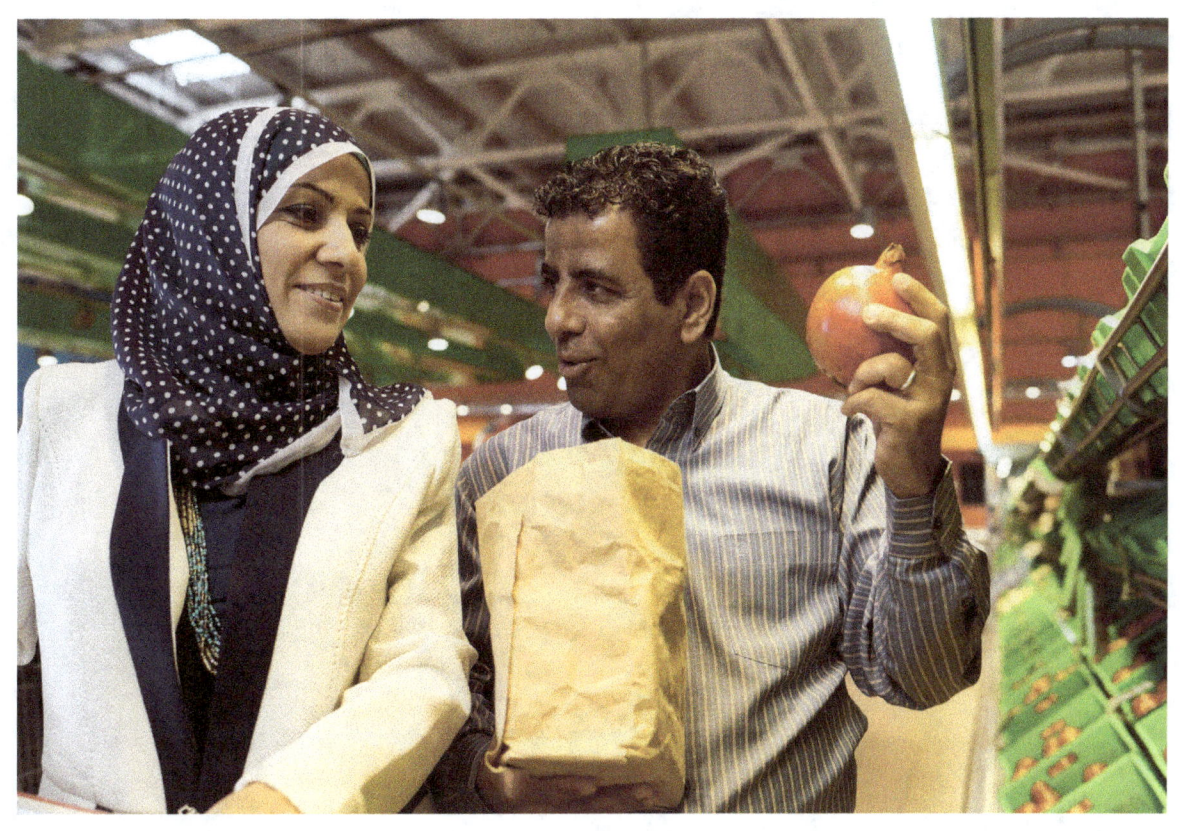

Benefits of pomegranate for men: fact or myth?

What are the benefits of pomegranate for men?
What do you need to know about it? What are the
general health benefits of pomegranate? The most
important information and details can be found in
.the following article

?Benefits of pomegranate for men: fact or myth
Let's learn about the benefits of pomegranate for
.men and some important information in this regard

Benefits of pomegranate for men
Pomegranate may carry many potential benefits for
men, here is a list of the most important ones

1. Treatment of erectile dysfunction

The use of pomegranate may help treat or reduce erectile dysfunction, and this is what studies say in this regard:

One study showed that drinking pomegranate juice regularly may help reduce or even treat erectile dysfunction, but it should be noted that this study was not conducted on humans.

A study conducted on a small group of men with erectile dysfunction showed that drinking pomegranate juice helped improve erection for some of them, but it should be noted that the sample on which this study was conducted was relatively small, and the results of the experiment are weak and insufficient. To settle the matter on the effectiveness of pomegranate juice in this regard.

So, although there are some preliminary studies indicating the existence of pomegranate benefits for men in this regard, the scientific evidence currently available is still inconclusive, and more research and studies are still needed to confirm or deny it

2. Prostate cancer resistance

One of the possible benefits of pomegranate for men is that it may help fight prostate cancer in several different ways, as pomegranate contains compounds that may help:

Inhibiting the spread and transmission of cancer cells, by weakening the links between these cells and some chemical signals that play a role in the spread of cancer cells.

Slowing down and inhibiting the growth of cancer cells, and increasing the rate of death of cancer cells, especially in men who are undergoing treatment for prostate cancer.

However, it must be noted that the benefits of pomegranate for men in this context are not confirmed yet.

3. Enhance sexual desire

Pomegranate fruits are an excellent source of antioxidants that may play an important role in improving reproductive health for both men and women, as the antioxidant content of pomegranate and some other important nutrients may help: lower cortisol levels and raise testosterone lev

So, because of the potential effect of pomegranate on the aforementioned hormones that play an important role in sexual health, especially testosterone, eating pomegranates may help boost vitality and improve libido in both men and women.

Health benefits of pomegranate
Pomegranate has other potential health benefits that may have a positive effect on both men and women, such as:

1. Improve the health of the circulatory system
Pomegranate contains a variety of nutrients that may have a role in improving the health of the circulatory system and reducing the chances of it developing diseases, such as heart attacks, due to the ability of these potential compounds to:

Reducing high blood pressure.
Reducing harmful and bad cholesterol, in exchange for increasing beneficial and good cholesterol

2. Treating anemia

Eating pomegranates or drinking pomegranate juice can help combat and treat anemia in several different ways, as follows:

Pomegranate may help maintain healthy blood circulation in various parts of the body.

Pomegranate may have a positive effect on anemia, as consuming iron-rich pomegranate may help relieve symptoms of anemia, such as: weakness, dizziness, and fatigue.

3. Improve bone and joint health

The delicious pomegranate fruit may have many potential benefits for bone health, as pomegranate is a good source of many nutrients that may contribute to relieving symptoms of some bone diseases, such as the following diseases: osteoporosis, arthritis, and osteoporosis. , and osteoarthritis.

The potential benefits of pomegranate in this regard are often attributed to the fact that it contains substances that may help reduce inflammation, which may play a role in exacerbating and worsening some of the aforementioned conditions

4. Additional benefits of pomegranate

Pomegranate can have many other potential benefits, such as:

Fighting some types of cancer, such as breast cancer.

Reducing the chances of mouth and teeth infection with some diseases and health problems.

Improving the health of the digestive system, and improving the condition of patients with some problems and diseases of the digestive system, such as: Crohn's disease and ulcerative colitis.

Other benefits, such as: improving and strengthening memory, improving athletic performance, reducing hair loss, and resisting signs of skin aging

Pomegranate damage

Here is a list of the most prominent potential harms of pomegranate:

Low blood pressure to levels that may be dangerous, especially in people with hypotension, and people who are about to undergo surgery of some kind.

The appearance of symptoms indicating an allergy to pomegranate, such as: breathing difficulties, vomiting, itching and red eyes.

Introducing large amounts of sugars to the body, especially when consuming pomegranate juice on a daily basis.

Possible complications when using pomegranate extract or when using other parts of pomegranate other than pulp, as pomegranate peels and roots may contain toxic substances.

A negative effect on the effect and mode of action of certain types of medicines when taking pomegranate with these medicines, such as blood-thinning medicines

Pomegranate damage

Here is a list of the most prominent potential harms of pomegranate:

Low blood pressure to levels that may be dangerous, especially in people with hypotension, and people who are about to undergo surgery of some kind.

The appearance of symptoms indicating an allergy to pomegranate, such as: breathing difficulties, vomiting, itching and red eyes.

Introducing large amounts of sugars to the body, especially when consuming pomegranate juice on a daily basis.

Possible complications when using pomegranate extract or when using other parts of pomegranate other than pulp, as pomegranate peels and roots may contain toxic substances.

A negative effect on the effect and mode of action of certain types of medicines when taking pomegranate with these medicines, such as blood-thinning medicines

Learn about the benefits of pomegranate for the heart

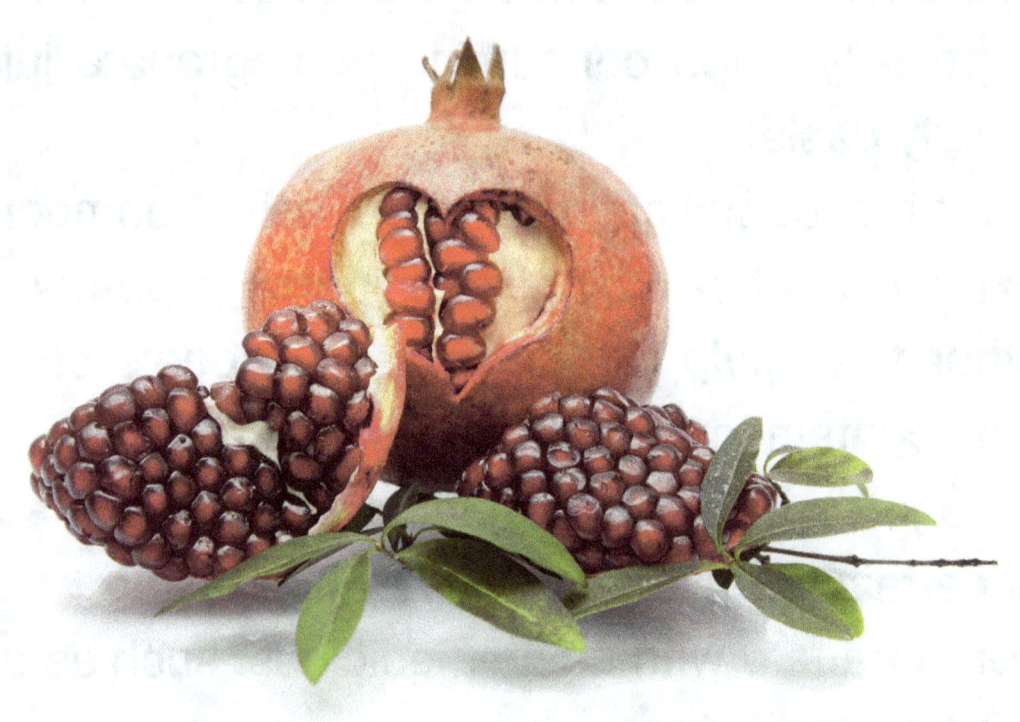

Benefits of pomegranate for the heart: get to know them

What is the truth about the benefits of pomegranate for the heart? And what is the recommended daily intake to reap the benefits it offers? We will learn about all that and more through this article.

Benefits of pomegranate for the heart: get to know them

Pomegranate is an excellent natural source of many nutrients, vitamins and minerals, but what are the benefits of pomegranate for the heart? What are its main benefits? Details in the following article

Benefits of pomegranate for the heart: is it real and exist?

The benefits of pomegranate for the heart can be explained by the following points:

1 – Pomegranate is an excellent source of antioxidants, especially polyphenols, as the percentage of antioxidants in it may reach three times those found in green tea, along with anthocyanins and tannins, this makes pomegranate ideal for preventing atherosclerosis And protect the heart by lowering blood cholesterol.

2– The antioxidants present in pomegranate help increase the activity of the Paraoxonase enzyme, which leads to the breakdown of harmful oxidized fats, and it also has an important role in lowering blood pressure levels.

3– Daily consumption of pomegranate may improve stress-induced myocardial ischemia in patients with coronary artery disease.

4Pomegranate contributes to reducing the severity and duration of angina pectoris in patients with myocardial ischemia

The recommended amount to obtain the benefits of pomegranate for the heart

It is recommended to eat approximately one and a half to two cups of pomegranate daily, which is equivalent to one and a half to two fruits. This ensures obtaining the dense nutrients present in the pomegranate without fear of consuming a high percentage of fat or calories, as one cup of it contains the equivalent of 174 calories. only.

General benefits of pomegranate

After we got to know the benefits of pomegranate for the heart, we must take a quick glance at the most important general benefits of pomegranate for the body, the most prominent of which include the following:

Provides the body with vitamin C: One pomegranate fruit may provide about 40% of the daily need for vitamin C.

Prevents cancer: Pomegranate may help stop the growth of prostate cancer cells, and it may contribute to reducing the risk of cancer

Protects against Alzheimer's: The antioxidants present in pomegranate may in turn help prevent memory impairment and Alzheimer's.

Beneficial for the digestive system: Pomegranate can help improve digestion and reduce intestinal inflammation, especially in people with ulcerative colitis, Crohn's disease, and inflammatory bowel diseases.

Fights Inflammation: The high concentration of antioxidants prevents oxidative stress and fights inflammation throughout the body.

Prevents arthritis: Flavonols help prevent infections that cause cartilage damage and joint inflammation. This contributes to reducing the risk of rheumatoid arthritis and osteoporosis.

Lowers blood pressure: Regular consumption of pomegranate may lower systolic blood pressure.

Boosts Immunity: Pomegranate contains vitamin C and vitamin E, along with other nutrients that boost the immune system, which fight infection and prevent disease, and it has been shown that pomegranate has a strong effect on killing bacteria and viruses

Provides the body with vitamins and minerals: Pomegranate is an excellent source of potassium, vitamin K, vitamin C, vitamin E, and folate.

Improves memory: Pomegranate can improve memory and learning ability.

Promotes sexual health: Pomegranate reduces oxidative stress, which affects fertility in women and sperm in men.

Improves sports performance: Pomegranate juice is one of the best energy-boosting sports drinks, especially if beetroot or cherry juice is added to it, as it has the effect of relieving pain and improving overall body strength.

Pomegranate damage

Pomegranate consumption is considered safe for most people, but some may experience some side effects, which include the following:

1- Itching.
2- Difficulty breathing.
3- Swelling
4-Runny nose

Benefits of pomegranate for women

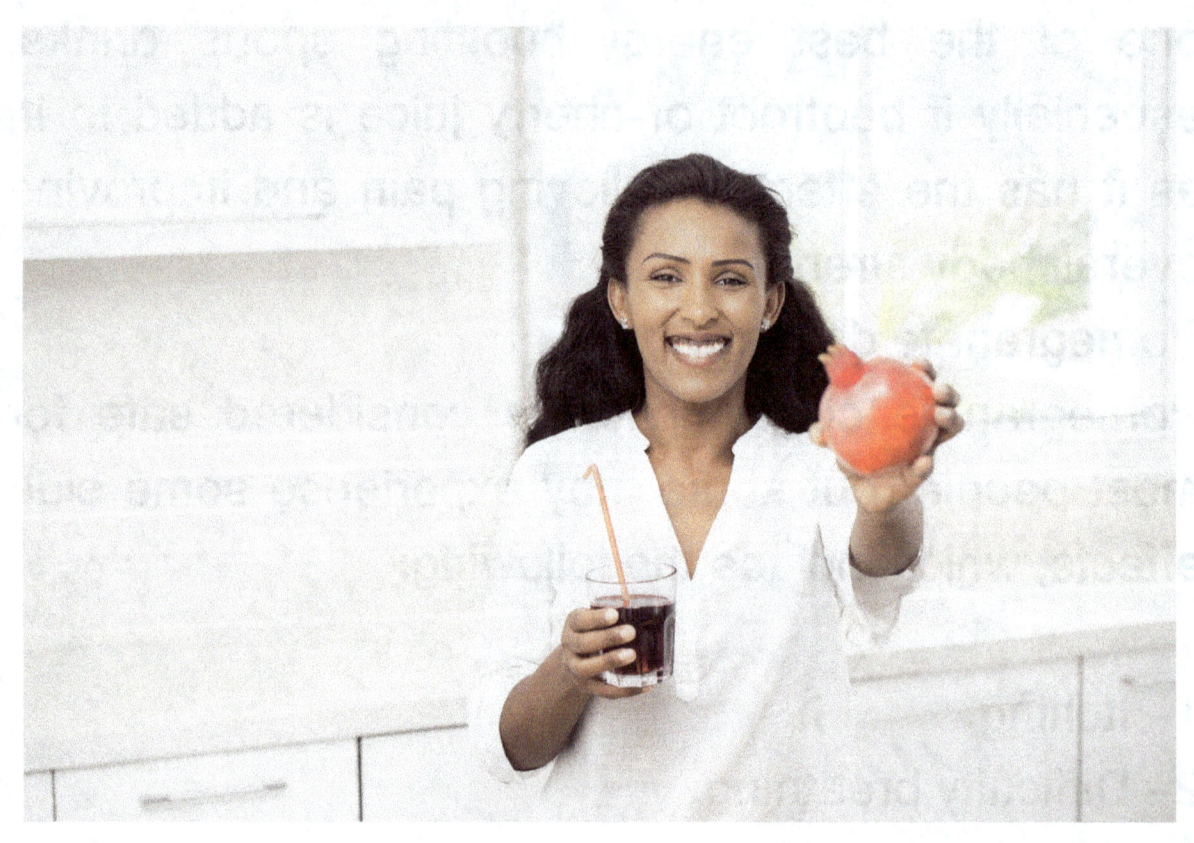

Benefits of pomegranate for women

Pomegranate has a delicious taste and offers many health benefits to the body. Is one of its health properties related to women's health in particular? Here is the most important information about the benefits of pomegranate for women.

Benefits of pomegranate for women

What are the benefits of pomegranate for women? Here are the most important details in the following article

Benefits of pomegranate for women

Pomegranate has properties related to sexual health and helps in treating infertility in women. It may also help protect the fetus from deformities, due to multiple reasons, including:

Contains phytoestrogens

Pomegranate seeds contain phytoestrogens that help prevent diseases and problems of the reproductive system in women, such as: uterine fibroids, endometriosis, uterine cancer, ovarian cancer, and breast cancer.

Contains folic acid

Pomegranate is one of the most important foods rich in folic acid, which in turn helps in the development and growth of the fetus and reduces malformations, especially malformations of the brain and spinal cord. Therefore, pomegranate is important for the health of a pregnant woman

Helps promote uterine health
Pomegranate helps increase blood flow to the uterus, thus maintaining its health and increasing the chances of successful fertilization and embryo adhesion to the lining of the uterus.

Contains flavanoids and antioxidants
Pomegranate is one of the richest foods in antioxidants that contribute to enhancing the health of the immune system, resisting diseases and infections, and reducing oxidative stress, thus helping to enhance the health of the reproductive system and fertility.

Raise the level of testosterone
Pomegranate may help raise the level of testosterone, and although it is a male hormone, its presence in appropriate quantities in a woman's body is important for several reasons, including: increasing sexual desire and improving fertility

The benefits of pomegranate for men and women
In addition to the benefits of pomegranate for women, here are the most important potential benefits of pomegranate for both sexes:

Rich in vitamins
Pomegranate is a rich source of vitamins, especially vitamin C, which may provide 40% of the body's need for vitamin C during the day.

It is also a source of vitamin E, vitamin K, folic acid, and potassium.

Promote digestion
Eating pomegranate may help reduce inflammation and improve digestion, especially in people who suffer from chronic diseases related to the digestive system, such as: Crohn's disease and ulcerative colitis.

However, please do not eat too much pomegranate if you have diarrhea. Because it may make things worse in that case

Promotes heart health

Pomegranate helps in promoting heart health, by increasing blood flow, preventing atherosclerosis and cholesterol accumulation, and helping to regulate diastolic blood pressure, thus preventing various heart diseases.

Relieve arthritis

Pomegranate has anti-inflammatory properties, especially related to joints, bones, and cartilage erosion. Therefore, it may contribute to relieving the pain of osteoarthritis, rheumatism, and any diseases related to arthritis.

Cancer prevention

Pomegranate has anti-cancer properties because it is rich in polyphenols, so that recent research studies the effect of pomegranate in the prevention and treatment of cancer, especially prostate cancer, kidney cancer, lung cancer, breast cancer, and cervical cancer.

It may also help limit the spread of cancer cells

Promotes oral and dental health

Pomegranate extracts may help reduce the growth of harmful bacteria in the mouth and reduce high acidity, thus preventing gum problems and diseases and tooth decay.

Other benefits of pomegranate

Here are some other potential benefits of pomegranate:

It possesses anti-bacterial properties.

It promotes healthy skin.

Helps regulate blood sugar.

Contributes to the prevention of Alzheimer's disease

Warnings about pomegranate

Pomegranate is a very safe food, but please pay attention to some warnings, including the following:

Please note that if you suffer from allergy to plants, the probability of allergy to pomegranate is high.

Please be careful if you suffer from low blood pressure, because pomegranate may increase the possibility of severe hypotension in this case.

Eating pomegranate in large quantities should be stopped at least two weeks before any surgery, due to its effect on blood pressure and the possibility of its interaction with antihypertensive drugs

Does pomegranate increase weight or lead to its decrease?

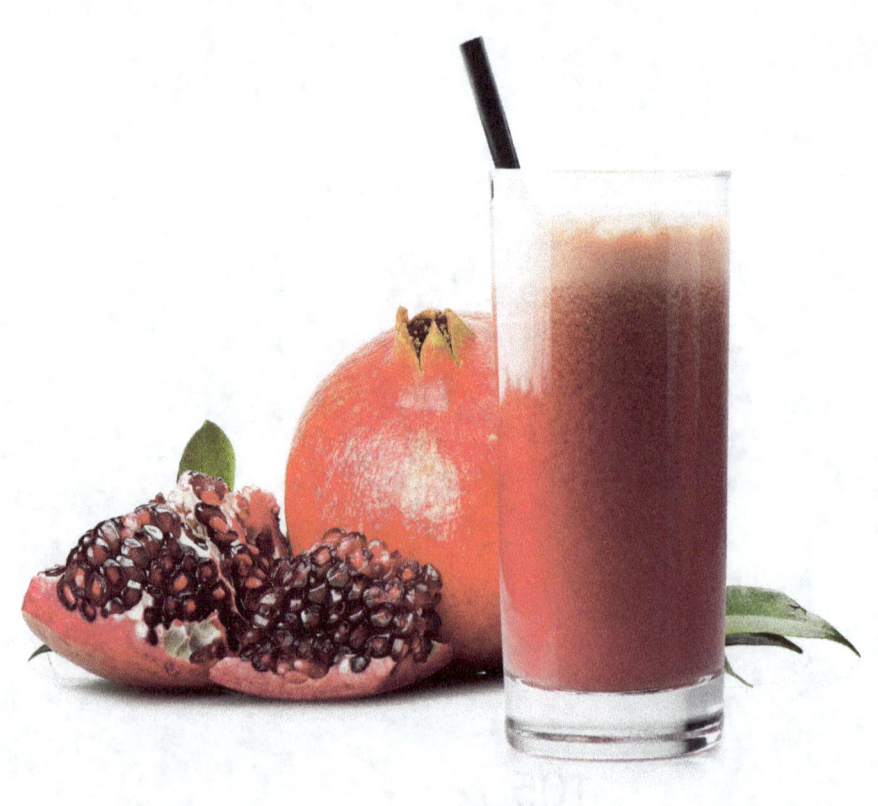

Does pomegranate increase weight or lead to its decrease?

Some people think that fruits contain an amount of sugars that lead to a significant increase in weight, but what about pomegranates? Does pomegranate increase weight?

Does pomegranate increase weight or lead to its decrease?
Pomegranate contains many important and beneficial elements for human health, but what is to be done if you follow a diet? Does pomegranate really make you gain weight

Does pomegranate increase weight or lead to its decrease?

Many people wonder about does pomegranate gain weight? So the answer is no, on the contrary, pomegranate helps to lose weight, especially when unhealthy food and drinks are replaced with pomegranate juice.

Pomegranate helps in losing weight and fighting excess obesity, as pomegranate contains many substances with antioxidant properties and polyphenols, which in turn help in losing weight.

How does pomegranate help in losing weight? After we got to know the answer to the question, does pomegranate increase weight? Here are some of the most important properties of pomegranate that help in losing weight significantly

1. Reducing fat and preventing insulin resistance
Pomegranate contains ellagic acid, which helps reduce body fat and increase insulin sensitivity and response.

The body's resistance to insulin is usually associated with weight gain, as pomegranate contains anthocyanin, which helps prevent the body's resistance to insulin.

Pomegranate also contains tannin and flavonoids that help fight obesity and gain weight.

2. Appetite control
Pomegranate is a rich source of fiber that gives the body a feeling of fullness and prevents a person from eating excessively unhealthy food, which helps in losing weight.

Where fiber is slowly absorbed into the body, which helps to feel full for long periods

3. Pomegranates are low in calories

100 grams of pomegranate contains 83 calories, and it does not contain any fat or cholesterol.

Pomegranate helps to give a person a feeling of satiety despite containing a few calories, especially when compared to eating hamburgers or pizza that contain double calories.

4. Pomegranate contains nutrients

Pomegranate contains many nutrients, such as: protein, fiber, vitamin C, vitamin K, vitamin B12, and folate, and one pomegranate contains five grams of protein.

The many nutrients found in pomegranate help fight obesity factors and reduce human weight

5. Fight against oxidative stress

Eating excessively unhealthy foods that cause obesity leads to an increase in oxidation factors within the body, as pomegranate contains many substances with antioxidant properties that help reduce the level of sugar in the body, cholesterol, and fats.

Antioxidants also help to lose weight and increase the body's metabolism rate

Tips that interest you about eating pomegranate

After clarifying whether pomegranate increases weight or leads to its decrease? And the properties of pomegranate that help in losing weight, here are some important tips:

Pomegranate can be added to many food ingredients in order to prepare various healthy dishes, and here are some of the ingredients to which pomegranate can be added in order to obtain a healthy and delicious mixture:

Buttermilk or Greek yogurt.

Oats.

quinoa grains

Cranberry sauce.

roasted carrots.

grilled chicken.

Fresh pomegranate juice can be made and replace all carbonated and sugary drinks. Care must be taken to choose only fresh pomegranate juice.

Pomegranate interacts with some medications just like grapefruit, so it is recommended to consult a doctor if it is consumed with various medications, as the interaction of pomegranate with medications sometimes increases the side effects of these medications, so consulting a doctor is essential

Pomegranate for pregnant women: damage and benefits

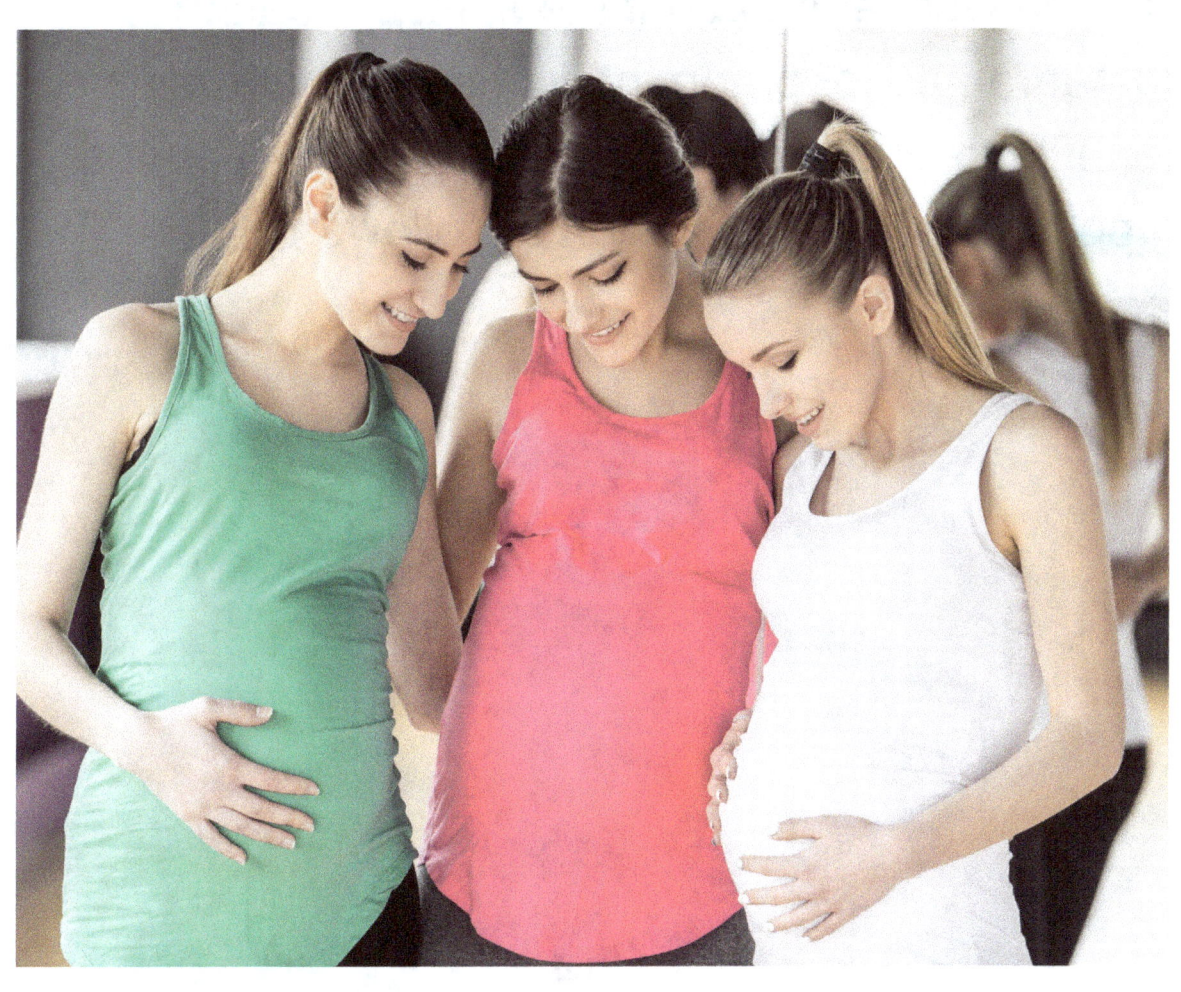

Pomegranate for pregnant women: damage and benefits

During pregnancy, a woman cares about the foods she eats so that it does not affect her and her fetus, and for this reason, we present to you the benefits of pomegranate for pregnant women.

Pomegranate for pregnant women: damage and benefits
Are you wondering about the safety of eating pomegranate for pregnant women? What are its benefits to you and your fetus? Here are the most important of this information as follows

Pomegranate for pregnant women: Is it safe?

In most cases, eating pomegranate and its juice is safe during pregnancy, but of course it is always preferable to consult your doctor who can assess your health condition.

Pomegranate should also be eaten in moderate quantities and according to important conditions, and clarification in the following:

It is advised to avoid pomegranate extract, which would increase uterine contractions, and to only eat fresh pomegranate or home-made juice.

It is preferable to eat pomegranates in moderation, as pomegranate juice is rich in calories, which increases weight.

It is recommended to consult a doctor if the pregnant woman is taking some medications, as pomegranate and its juice may interact with some medications, causing health problems

Benefits of pomegranate for pregnant women
Pomegranate is rich in various nutrients, which are beneficial for you and your fetus if consumed in moderate amounts, while pomegranate juice is a good way to keep your body hydrated.

The benefits of pomegranate for pregnant women are divided into two parts, which are as follows:

1. The benefits of pomegranate seeds for pregnant women
Pomegranate seeds contain many of the following nutrients, which provide many benefits for pregnant women:

Dietary fiber
Pomegranate is rich in dietary fiber, which means that half a cup of pomegranate seeds contains approximately 5 grams of fiber, which has many health benefits

During pregnancy, pregnant women suffer in particular from constipation and various digestive problems, but eating pomegranate helps protect you from this injury, as the fibers move the intestines and relieve you of discomfort.

According to the American Pregnancy Association, pregnant women need 25-30 grams of dietary fiber per day.

Iron

Pomegranate is one of the most iron-rich foods, and this is one of the minerals that a pregnant woman needs during her pregnancy.

Not getting enough iron increases your risk of anemia, and thus many health complications. Pregnant women who suffer from anemia are more likely to give birth prematurely.

It is possible that the doctor advises you to take iron supplements, on the other hand, eating pomegranate for pregnant women would reflect positively on iron levels as well.

vitamin C

Pomegranate is a good source of vitamin C, which enhances the absorption of iron into your body

2. Benefits of pomegranate juice for pregnant women

The benefits of pomegranate for a pregnant woman are not limited to eating it only, but its juice would provide you with the following elements, which are followed by many benefits:

Calories

During pregnancy, you need 2,000–2,200 calories per day in the second and third trimesters, so consuming 230 milliliters of pomegranate juice provides you with 136 calories, which is good for you.

folate

You need folate during pregnancy, as it is necessary and important for the growth of your fetus. One serving of pomegranate juice provides you with 60 milligrams of folate.

The recommended daily intake of folate during pregnancy is 600 milligrams, but not less than 400 milligrams per day.

Getting the right amount of folate means normal growth for your fetus and protecting it from various birth defects

Vitamin K

One serving of pomegranate juice contains 26.1 micrograms of vitamin K, and pregnant women need 90 micrograms of it daily.

Vitamin K supports the growth and development of your baby's bones and protects you from blood clots during pregnancy.

potassium

230 milliliters of pomegranate juice contains 538 milligrams of potassium, which is important for you during pregnancy, so pomegranate for pregnant women contributes to preventing you from getting foot cramps, which are famous during this period, and also contributes to treating them.

Antioxidants

Antioxidants have many different health benefits, they protect your placenta from damage and various infections, and they also provide the necessary protection for the brain of the fetus

Pomegranate and skin: benefits and recipes

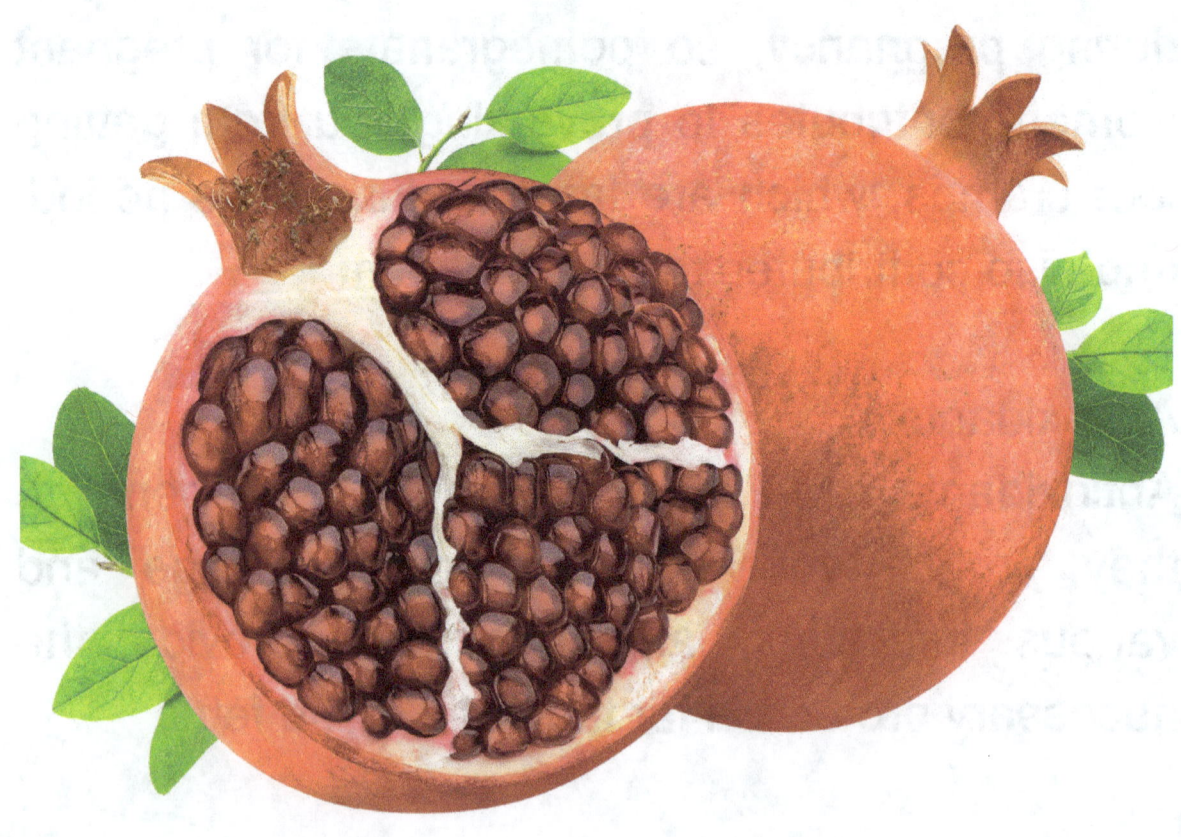

Pomegranate and skin: benefits and recipes

Do you want to protect your skin from harmful UV rays in a natural way? If you really want to, enjoy the many benefits of pomegranate for the skin in the following ways:

Pomegranate and skin: benefits and recipes
Pomegranate contains a lot of nutrients, which makes it really important for improving your health from the inside and outside. Learn about the most important benefits of pomegranate for the skin, and some of the ways to use it in the following

Benefits of pomegranate for the skin

There are several benefits of pomegranate for skin health, including:

1. Reducing skin inflammation

Pomegranate contains antioxidants that may help reduce the effects of free radical damage and skin infections.

Antioxidants may be able to reduce the symptoms of some common skin conditions, such as acne and eczema.

2. Protecting epidermal cells

Some of the antioxidants found in pomegranate, such as vitamin C, reduce cell damage in your body.

Eating pomegranate seeds can be useful for cell regeneration, but applying it topically may ensure that you get better results for its benefits on the skin

3. Prevention of aging

Studies conducted on a group of mice whose skin was applied pomegranate peel oil indicated that the antioxidants in this oil helped reduce wrinkle spots and ageing, but did not prevent them completely.

The effects of the antioxidants are thought to contribute to increased cell turnover, which enables your skin to shed old skin cells.

4. Getting rid of germs

Pomegranate contains natural antibacterials that may help get rid of harmful bacteria and fungi from your skin.

These benefits of applying pomegranate to the skin may really help treat acne-causing bacteria, and get rid of skin spots.

5. UV protection

The antioxidants in pomegranate have also been shown to help provide the skin with natural protection against UV rays.

It is worth noting that despite the benefits of pomegranate for the skin in preventing harmful rays, you still have to use daily sunscreen

6. Exfoliate the skin naturally

Regular exfoliation helps get rid of dead skin cells, which reduces the appearance of blemishes, acne, and signs of skin aging.

These benefits are directly related to the benefits of pomegranate on the skin when ground pomegranate seeds are applied to the skin.

Ways to use pomegranate for the skin

There are many ways to benefit from the benefits of pomegranate for the skin, by adding it to some food dishes or drinking its juice, and you can also use pomegranate in the following way:

Natural exfoliator

If you can't find a good exfoliator, why not try some pomegranate seeds? You can follow these steps:

1- Grind pomegranate seeds and apply it on the skin, it will release all the nutrients on your skin, nourishing it from the outside.

2- Make sure to wash your face well after exfoliating, and apply your moisturizing cream.

3- Use a pomegranate scrub for your skin once or twice a week to remove dead skin cells

Pomegranate peel oil

The benefits of pomegranate can be obtained in this case through pomegranate peel oil that is purchased from pharmacies or popular markets:

1- Use pomegranate peel oils as a skin softener by applying them before using moisturizing ointments.
2- Massage your skin with pomegranate peel oil twice a day to get the best results.

pomegranate supplements

Pomegranate is also available in the form of capsules and tablets, which are often sold in pharmacies.

Instead of applying pureed pomegranate or pomegranate peel oil to the skin topically, you can take these supplements orally.

Talk to your doctor before use, and be sure to take your supplements as directed

Side effects of pomegranate on the skin
After getting to know the benefits of pomegranate for the skin, we note that it may cause some side effects, including the following:

Applying pomegranate or its oil to the skin may cause some irritation, sensitivity and redness, so we advise you to test the pomegranate on a small part of the skin before applying it to the facial skin. The pomegranate peel may scratch the skin, so make sure to grind the seeds well and apply the peel in gentle, circular motions

Pomegranate mask types and benefits

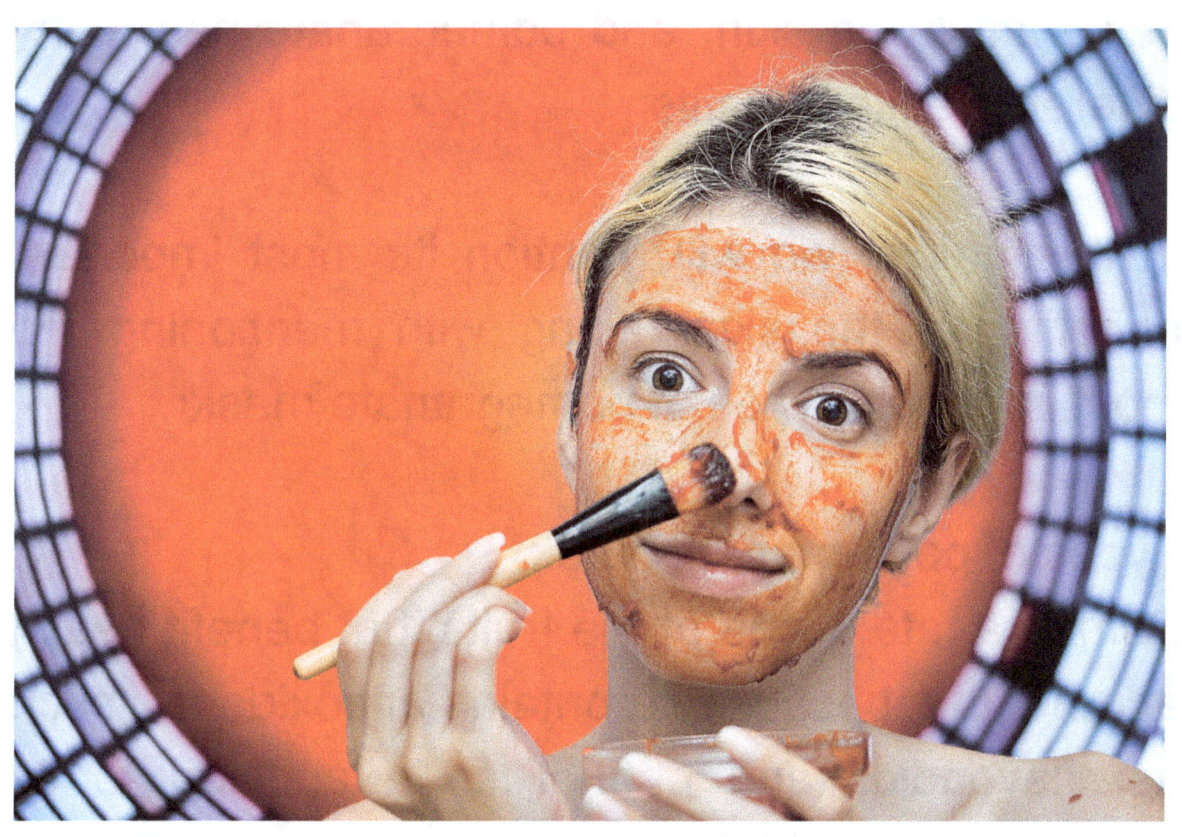

Pomegranate mask: types and benefits

Pomegranate has many diverse health benefits, especially for the skin, and in this article we will mention the most important types of pomegranate mask used.

Pomegranate mask: types and benefits
Pomegranate (Pomegranate) is a sweet fruit that has a thick red skin, and pomegranate has many different health benefits.

In this article, we will mention its most important benefits for the skin, along with mentioning the most important types of pomegranate mask:

Types of pomegranate mask
Pomegranate is one of the fruits that benefit health and beauty, because it contains antioxidants, such as: flavonoids and phenolics, in addition to its richness in vitamin E, vitamin A, and vitamin C

Therefore, the use of a pomegranate mask can play a major role in giving the individual smooth and glowing skin, and this fruit has the ability to help produce collagen, which helps in the process of tightening the skin.

There are many types of pomegranate mask used, based on the benefit that the individual will obtain through its application, and we will now mention the most important types of these pomegranate masks, with mentioning the benefit that is associated with this mask:

1. Pomegranate and lemon mask

The benefit of applying the pomegranate and lemon mask lies in the treatment of tanning that some individuals may suffer from. Here are the steps to prepare this mask:

the components

Among the most important components used in applying this type of mask are the following:

One tablespoon of pomegranate paste.

One teaspoon of lemon juice

How to use

Which is done by following:

1– The above ingredients are mixed together.

2– Apply this mask to the face and neck.

3– Leave it on the skin for at least 30 minutes.

4– After that, wash your face with water.

5– It is recommended to apply this mask two or three times per week.

2. Pomegranate and papaya mask

Which is used in order to obtain fresh and glowing skin, and it can be prepared through the following:

the components

Among its most important components are the following:

Two tablespoons of pomegranate seed oil.

One tablespoon of green papaya powder.

One teaspoon of grape seed oil.

One teaspoon of grape seeds

How to use

This is done by following all of the following:

1- Mix all the previously mentioned ingredients together well.

2- Apply this prepared mixture on the face.

3- Leave it on the face for at least 30 minutes.

4- Wash it with cold water.

5- This process is repeated twice during one week

3. Pomegranate and green tea mask

Pomegranate and green tea mask is usually used to treat acne that some individuals may suffer from sometimes, and it can be prepared as follows:

the components

Among its most important components:

One tablespoon of pomegranate paste.

A tablespoon of milk.

One tablespoon of green tea.

One tablespoon of honey

How to use

As for the method of using it, it is done by following the following:

1- Mix all the above ingredients together in a bowl.

2- Apply this mixture on the face and massage for at least 5-10 minutes.

3- Leave this paste on the face for 20 minutes.

4- Wash it after that with cold water.

5- This type of mask should be applied twice a week

Benefits of pomegranate mask for the skin

Pomegranate mask has many benefits for the skin, the most important of which are the following:

Prevention and prevention of premature aging.

Moisturizing dry and irritated skin.

Prevention of acne and some other types of pimples, in addition to its ability to control excess oil on the skin.

Treat and heal scars.

Skin tightening, reducing the appearance of lines and wrinkles on the skin.

Skin cancer prevention

Side effects of pomegranate mask

Despite the inherent benefits of pomegranate mask, it is like other fruits that may have some side effects, and the most prominent of these effects are the following:

Suffering from pomegranate allergy and itching.
swelling.
Runny nose.
Difficulty breathing.
Interactions that may occur with some types of drugs, sometimes causing some serious harm to the individual

Pomegranate for infants: between benefits and harms

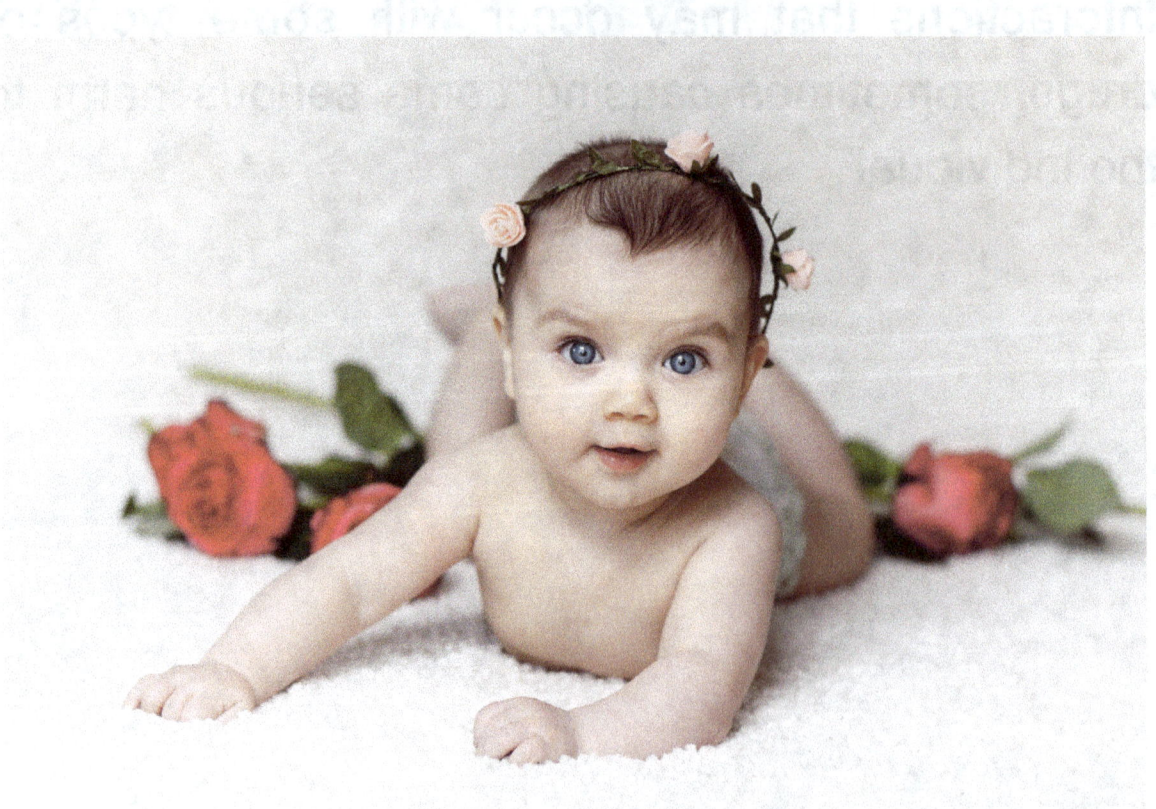

Pomegranate for infants: between benefits and harms

What are the benefits of pomegranate for infants? And when can it be introduced to infants? And what are the methods of preparing it, in addition to the precautions that must be taken into account? Here are the details in this article.

Pomegranate for infants: between benefits and harms

Pomegranate includes high levels of vitamins and minerals that ensure that the child gets the natural nutrients he needs, and to include pomegranate for infants in their diet, we must share some of the information you need about it. More information about pomegranate for infants in the following article

Pomegranate for infants: benefits

Pomegranate may provide the following benefits to infants:

1. Build the immune system

The child may be exposed to frequent cold and cough problems, and pomegranate can help alleviate this problem and prevent infection, as it is rich in vitamin C and vitamin E, which play an important role in building the immune system and fighting inflammation and infection, and in addition to that, it also includes a group of minerals such as iron, potassium and folate, which It also has the same role.

2. Fighting bacterial infection

Pomegranate contains antioxidants and biochemical enzymes that help reduce and fight bacterial infections.

3. Improve digestion

Pomegranate may help treat digestive problems such as dysentery, diarrhea, vomiting, constipation, and dysentery, thanks to its fiber content

4. Elimination of intestinal worms

Intestinal worms are a common problem in children, and they multiply either in the small or large intestine. It is believed that pomegranate, thanks to its anti-helminthic properties, may fight these parasites and prevent their re-establishment.

Intestinal worms or parasites reside in either the small or large intestine and reproduce by feeding on nutrients, and pomegranate juice is a great antidote for killing these worms.

5. Fighting a fever

Pomegranate is one of the natural remedies for fever, as it provides the body with nutrients that lower the high body temperature, which the body lacks during a fever.

6. Fight cold and cough

Thanks to its antioxidant properties, pomegranate helps fight cold and cough, especially when ginger and black pepper are added to it

Pomegranate for infants: when can it be introduced to infants?

Pomegranate is considered one of the fruits that are safe to be presented to the child after reaching the age of six months, and it can be presented to the child in several different ways, with the need to prepare it in a way that suits the age of the child. And if the child cannot eat these seeds, it is recommended to get rid of them completely.

Pomegranate for infants: method of preparation

You can easily prepare pomegranate and serve it to the infant by following simple steps that are summarized as follows:

Pomegranate juice for infants

Follow these steps to prepare it:

1- Extract the pomegranate seeds from the fruit and make sure that they are free of white pulp.

2- Put the pomegranate in the juicer and blend it well until it becomes liquid.

3- Purify pomegranate juice from impurities, and initially give it to the child in small quantities

Pomegranate puree for infants

Follow these steps to prepare it:

1- Extract the pomegranate seeds from the fruit and make sure that they are free of white pulp.

2- Put the pomegranate in a blender, add a little water or pomegranate juice to it and mix well to get a smooth puree.

3- Add more liquids when mixing in case the puree has a thick consistency to suit the child's age.

Pomegranate for infants: precautions

Below is a set of precautions that must be taken into account when offering pomegranate to infants:

Do not offer pomegranate seeds directly to the infant, but rather prepare it in the form of puree or juice until he is able to eat solid foods.

Avoid leaving the white pulp of the fruit while preparing the pomegranate for the baby; Because its taste will not be palatable to him.

Offer about 1/4 - 1/2 cup of pomegranate juice or puree to the child; Because excessive consumption will expose him to the problem of nausea and diarrhea.

Avoid offering pomegranate to the child before bedtime. Because it may cause him dental problems

Benefits of pomegranate for children: Learn about the most famous

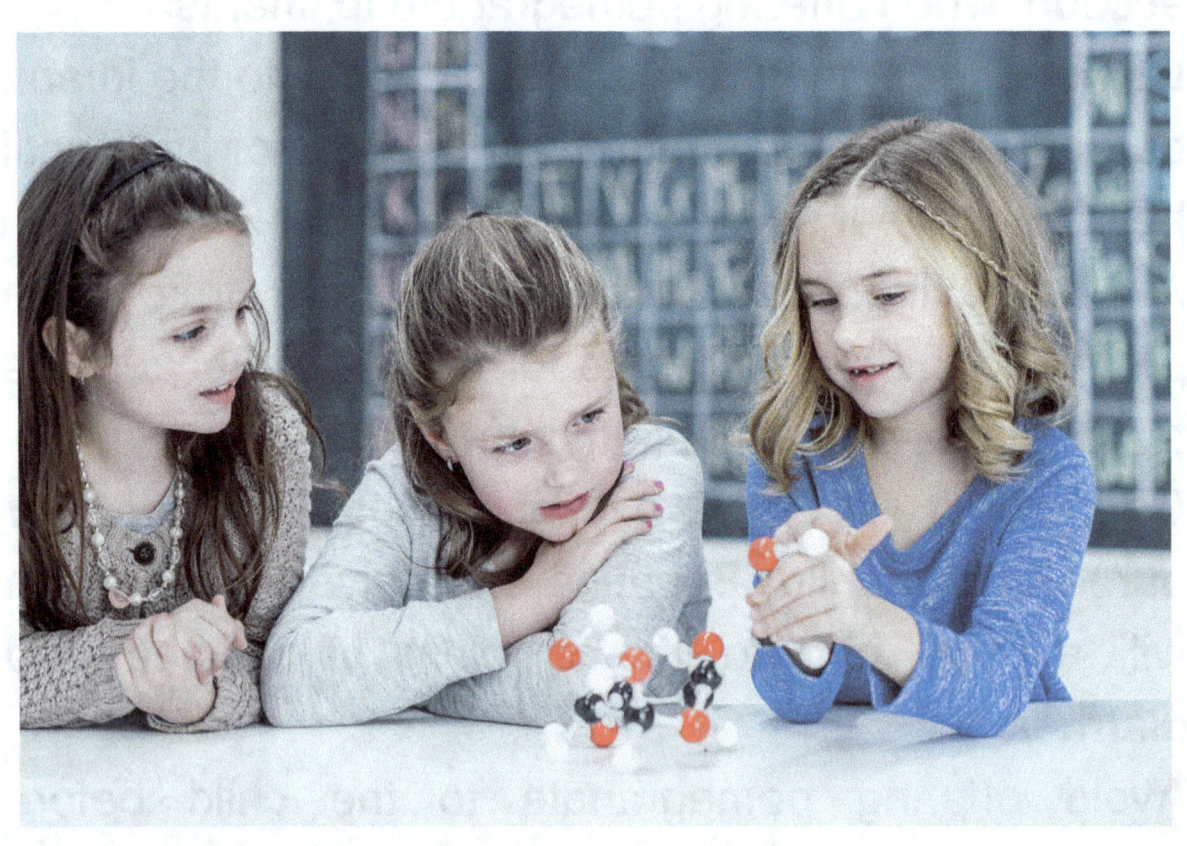

Benefits of pomegranate for children: Learn about the most famous

Pomegranate is one of the favorite fruits for many individuals and for different age groups, as its rich content of beneficial and necessary nutrients makes it have many health benefits, so what are the most important benefits of pomegranate for children?

Benefits of pomegranate for children: Learn about the most famous
Pomegranate is a tropical fruit that contains large quantities of edible seeds. It is rich in nutrients that are beneficial for children in particular, as it works to promote health since their growing age. This fruit contains many vitamins such as vitamin A, vitamin C, and others

Here are the most important benefits of pomegranate for children:

Benefits of pomegranate for children
There are many potential nutritional health benefits of pomegranate for children in particular, and among the most important and prominent benefits of pomegranate for children are the following:

1. Boost immunity
Pomegranate is rich in vitamin C, which helps the body develop immunity and fight various infections. Eating it regularly and continuously may help reduce children's infection with colds and coughs.

2. Fighting bacterial infections
The benefits of pomegranate for children lie in the fact that it contains biochemical enzymes that work to reduce infections that the child may be exposed to, by destroying bacterial infections

3. Reducing digestive problems

In the past, the pomegranate fruit was used in some traditional medical practices, the most important of which is the treatment of various digestive problems, for example: constipation, diarrhea, and vomiting.

Pomegranate juice is one of the most effective juices in treating vomiting and resisting bacteria that cause diarrhea in children, and this has been proven through some clinical studies.

4. Fighting intestinal worms

Intestinal worms are parasites that live in the small or large intestine and multiply by feeding on certain nutrients. Pomegranate fruit has anthelmintic properties that help kill these intestinal worms.

This benefit of pomegranate benefits for children has been proven by doing some studies and clinical trials.

5. Prevention of fever

Pomegranate juice has the ability to control the fever that a child may suffer from, in addition to providing the body with some important nutrients that help reduce and prevent fever in the first place

6. Other benefits

Among the other potential benefits that can be included in the benefits of pomegranate for children are the following:

Treating dental problems.
Dysentery treatment.
Maintaining a healthy liver

Pomegranate precautions for children

Despite the many benefits of pomegranate for children, it is one of the fruits that must be adhered to with cautions presented to them, as eating it may result in some harm and risks, and the most prominent of these precautions are the following:

Stripping the pulp from the seeds before serving them to children, due to the possibility that the child may suffocate because of them in some cases.

Offer its juice first without the seeds, especially if the child will be eating this fruit for the first time.

Offer it on its own without combining it with any type of fruit or other food, in order to know immediately if the child has an allergic reaction to this type of fruit.

Strip it of the white skin when served as juice, as it will make the juice sour.

Avoid serving it before bed, as it may cause some dental problems.

It is used in the quantities recommended for children, because its excessive consumption may lead to diarrhea in the child, and the amount that is usually allowed does not exceed approximately 118-177 milliliters

Benefits of pomegranate juice before bed

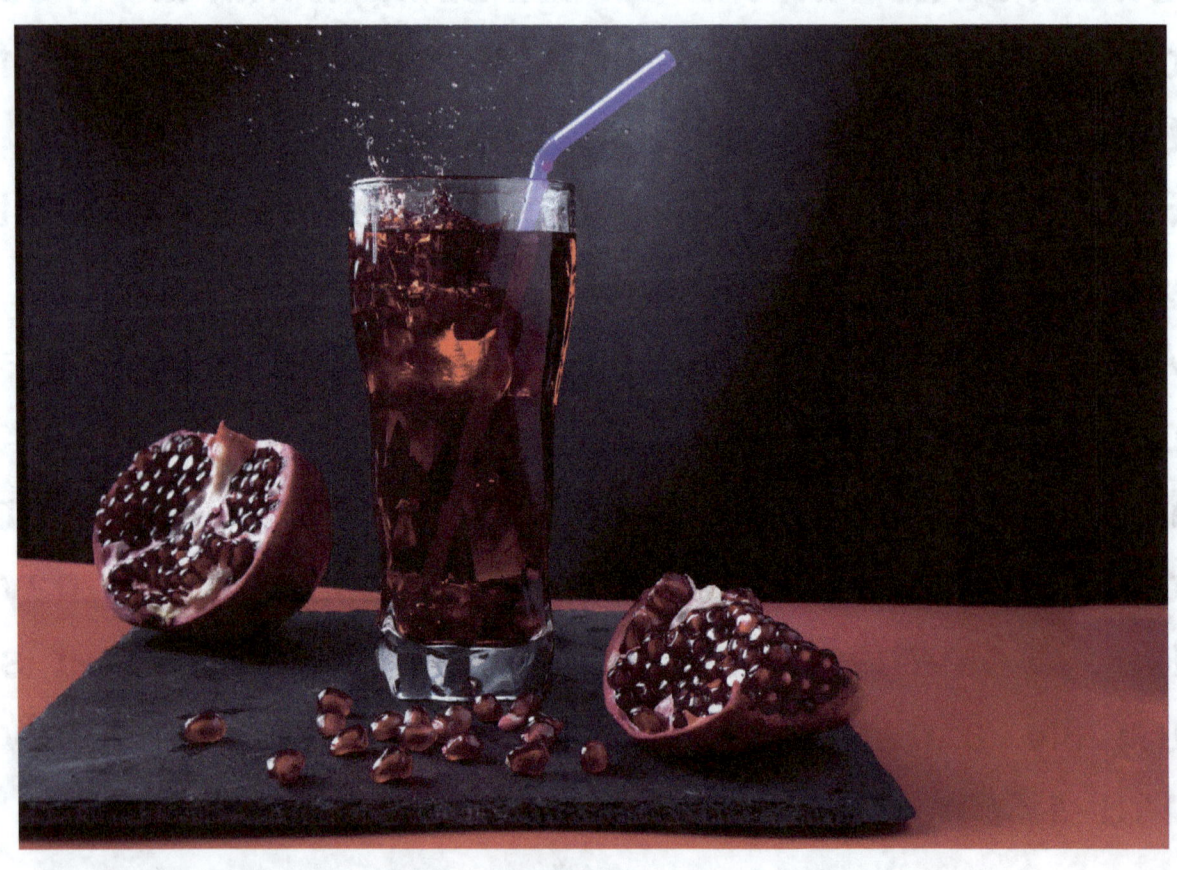

Benefits of pomegranate juice before bed

Pomegranate juice has been used as a remedy against many diseases since ancient times, but is consuming pomegranate juice really beneficial? What are the benefits of pomegranate juice before bed?

Benefits of pomegranate juice before bed
Pomegranate is one of the most beneficial fruits. Because it contains many compounds that benefit the body with great benefit, and in the following article we will learn about some of the benefits of pomegranate juice before bed

Benefits of pomegranate juice before bed

Pomegranate juice offers many potential benefits to the body, and among the benefits of pomegranate juice before bed, we mention:

1. Maintaining the health of the circulatory system

One of the benefits of pomegranate juice before bed is to maintain the health of the circulatory system. Pomegranate contains Punicalagins and Ellagitannins, which protect blood vessels from cholesterol deposits, and reduce the level of triglycerides and harmful blood cholesterol.

Pomegranate juice also helps lower systolic blood pressure, and reduce the risk of heart attacks and strokes. Because it contains Punicic acid.

2. Promote sexual health

Promoting sexual health is one of the benefits of pomegranate juice before bedtime, as pomegranate treats sperm dysfunction in men and treats infertility in women, and it also raises testosterone levels, which raises sex drive, and pomegranate also promotes blood flow in the body, which contributes to In the treatment of erectile dysfunction in men (Erectile Dysfunction)

3. Fighting different types of infections

One of the benefits of pomegranate juice before bed is fighting bacterial, fungal, and viral infections such as gingivitis and stomatitis. Pomegranate contains a number of vitamins that boost the body's immunity, such as: Vitamin C and Vitamin E.

Pomegranate juice also fights free radicals and inflammatory diseases. Because pomegranate contains the compound punicalagin, which provides anti-inflammatory properties, and among the inflammatory diseases that pomegranate juice helps to cure, we mention inflammatory bowel disease.

4. Protection against cancer

Protection against cancer is one of the benefits of pomegranate juice before bedtime, as it inhibits the growth of cancer cells and stimulates their death. Among the most important types of cancer that pomegranate juice fights is breast cancer and prostate cancer

5. Other benefits

Among the other benefits of pomegranate juice before bed, we mention:

Enhance verbal and visual memory.

Arthritis treatment.

Chronic obstructive pulmonary disease treatment.

Fight Alzheimer's disease and slow its progression.

Pomegranate juice damage before bed

After getting acquainted with a number of the benefits of pomegranate juice before bed, we have to identify some of its potential harms, as it may cause allergies in some people, and among the symptoms of pomegranate allergy we mention:

Feeling itchy in the body.

urticaria;

Swelling of the face, mouth and tongue.

Throat blockage and difficulty breathing

Special tips to drink pomegranate juice before bed

Despite the many benefits of pomegranate juice before going to bed, it is necessary to consult a specialist doctor before starting to consume pomegranate or its juice periodically. As pomegranate may interact with some medications, leading to many problems, such as: muscular disorders, rhabdomyolysis, and kidney failure.

Pomegranate may cause an increase in the concentration of drugs in the human body, which increases the risk of developing various symptoms of these drugs, and among the drugs that may interact with pomegranate juice, we mention:

1- Cholesterol-lowering drugs: such as Rosuvastatin.

2- Antiarrhythmic drugs: such as amiodarone and quinidine.

3- Calcium channel blockers: Felodipine and Nisoldipine.

4- Immunosuppressants: such as cyclosporine and tacrolimus.

4- Protease inhibitors: such as saquinavir

Pomegranate juice for anemia

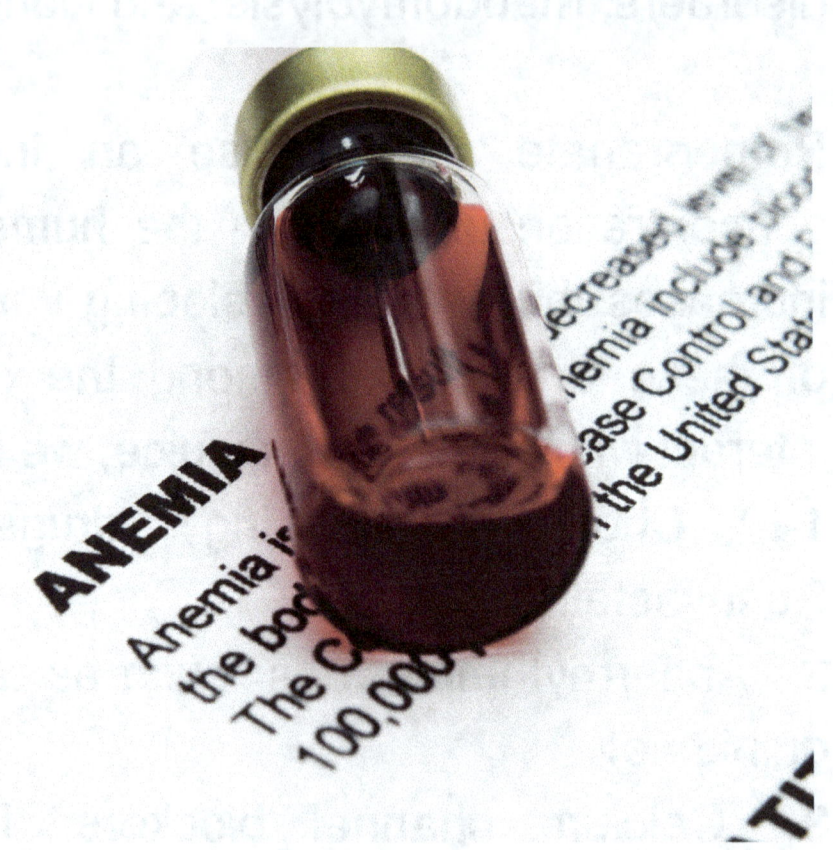

Pomegranate juice for anemia

What is the truth about the benefits of pomegranate juice for anemia? How can it be prepared? Follow the article to find out the answer.

Pomegranate juice for anemia

Anemia is a common problem, in which the blood does not contain enough healthy red blood cells to carry sufficient amounts of oxygen to the tissues of the body. In this article, we will present to you the truth about the benefits of pomegranate juice for anemia

Benefits of pomegranate juice for anemia: fact or myth?

Before talking about the benefits of pomegranate juice for anemia, it is necessary to define the problem of anemia, which is a common problem associated with a deficiency of hemoglobin in the body, which is a protein rich in iron that carries oxygen from the lungs to all cells of the body, and carbon dioxide from parts of the body to the lungs to get rid of it.

And now we will move on to the benefits of pomegranate juice for anemia. Pomegranate is one of the highly recommended fruits in cases of anemia, due to its richness in vitamin C, which contributes to enhancing the absorption of iron, as the body absorbs only 3% of the iron consumed through the intestines, and the existing vitamin C helps In pomegranate the body absorbs iron, because it is part of its metabolism

Pomegranate is also a rich source of iron, vitamin A, vitamin E, vitamin K, calcium, potassium, protein, fiber and many other nutrients. A healthy diet plays a role in increasing and maintaining hemoglobin levels, so regular consumption of pomegranate helps to increase Hemoglobin levels and fight anemia

Pomegranate juice for anemia: how to prepare it

Here are ways to prepare pomegranate juice for anemia:

Pomegranate juice for anemia

Pomegranate juice can be prepared as follows:

1- Prepare 5-6 pomegranates.

2- Remove the top part of the pomegranate peel, which is the part that looks like a crown.

3- Cut the pomegranate into several sections, you can divide it into 4 sections or more.

4- Fill a bowl with cold water, and separate the pomegranate seeds from the skin. This helps prevent the pomegranate juice from flowing everywhere.

5- Drain the water from the pomegranate seeds after peeling them all.

6- Put the pomegranate seeds in a blender, and blend it well for 15-20 seconds.

7 Pour the juice into a strainer, and use a rubber spatula to speed it up, as the juice is very thick and will take time to filter.

8- Pour the juice into serving cups. 5-6 pomegranates should yield 4 cups of juice

Pomegranate and beetroot juice for anemia
To prepare this juice, follow these steps:

1- Prepare the following ingredients: a fresh aloe vera leaf, 1/2 cup of chopped beetroot, 2 cups of pomegranate juice prepared in the previous recipe, and 1/4 teaspoon of black pepper.

2- Gently peel an aloe vera leaf, and take 2 tablespoons of pure aloe vera gel.

3- Add the pomegranate and beetroot juice to the food processor and mix well.

3- Add aloe vera gel and mix a little.

4- Add some black pepper and serve the juice

Warnings and harms of eating pomegranate juice

In general, pomegranate is safe to use for most people, and eating it in moderation does not cause any harm, but some may suffer from an allergy to it that causes the following symptoms to appear when eating pomegranate or its juice: itching, swelling, runny nose, and difficulty breathing, and some suffer from side effects in The digestive system when eating pomegranate or its juice, such as diarrhea.

On the other hand, it is advised to avoid eating some foods with pomegranate juice to treat anemia, such as: spinach, chocolate, tea, coffee, and alcohol, because they contain compounds that prevent iron absorption, and it is advised to maintain a time interval of at least 30 minutes between consuming pomegranate juice. And between these foods to ensure maximum iron absorption

Benefits of pomegranate on an empty stomach

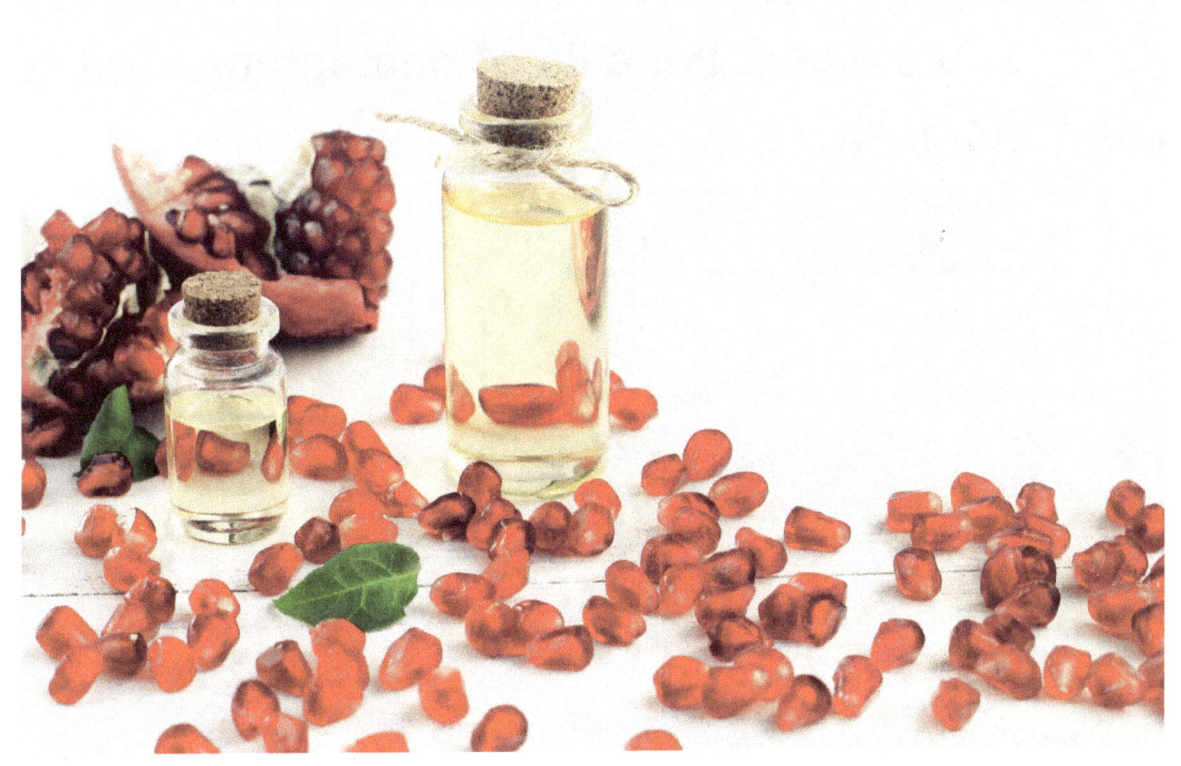

Benefits of pomegranate on an empty stomach

Eating pomegranate daily in your diet will make you gain many health benefits. Learn about the benefits of pomegranate on an empty stomach now.

Benefits of pomegranate on an empty stomach Pomegranate contains many useful plant compounds, which are unparalleled in other foods, and although the pomegranate peel is thick and inedible, there are hundreds of seeds inside that are edible directly, or in the form of juice. Here are the most prominent benefits of pomegranate on an empty stomach

Benefits of pomegranate on an empty stomach

Although there are no studies proving the benefits of pomegranates on an empty stomach in particular, there is a lot of research that has shown the health benefits of pomegranates, including the following:

1. It contains antioxidant compounds

Pomegranate seeds get their brilliant red color from powerful antioxidant polyphenols, which can help scavenge free radicals, preventing cell damage and reducing inflammation.

2. Prevents cancer

One of the benefits of pomegranate on an empty stomach is that it may help prevent certain types of cancer, as preliminary studies indicate that pomegranate juice can be beneficial for patients with prostate cancer, which may prevent the spread of cancer and reduce the possibility of death.

Laboratory studies also suggest that pomegranate extract can help fight breast cancer cells, but human studies are needed

3. Anti-inflammatory

Pomegranate is characterized by its ability to resist inflammation that it acquires from containing vitamin C, and therefore it may help protect against many common diseases, such as: certain types of cancer and type 2 diabetes, and thus the importance and benefits of pomegranate lie on an empty stomach.

4. Helps reduce blood pressure

One of the possible benefits of pomegranates on an empty stomach is that the antioxidants present in pomegranates may help reduce high blood pressure, which helps maintain good functioning of the arteries, heart and brain.

5. Fights arthritis

The flavanols in pomegranate juice may contribute to preventing the inflammation that causes osteoarthritis and cartilage damage, but studies are still ongoing to confirm the potential benefits of pomegranate juice for osteoporosis, rheumatoid arthritis, and other types of arthritis

6. Protection from heart disease

Many human studies have shown that pomegranate can protect against heart disease, as it lowers bad cholesterol, protects it from oxidative damage, and reduces triglycerides.

7. Fights bacterial infections and fungi

One of the main benefits of pomegranate on an empty stomach is that it fights bacteria, fungi, and viruses, which may help prevent common gum diseases and fungal infections.

8. Revitalizing memory and fighting Alzheimer's disease

A recent study revealed that consuming 248 grams (approximately 8 ounces) of pomegranate juice on a daily basis can improve learning and memory, and it is believed that the antioxidants present in pomegranates in high concentrations can help stop the progression of Alzheimer's disease and protect memory.

9. Rich in vitamins

One pomegranate juice contains more than 40% of the body's daily vitamin C needs, in addition to vitamin C and vitamin E. Pomegranate juice is also a good source of folate, potassium, and vitamin K

Pomegranate damage to the stomach: do you outweigh its benefits?

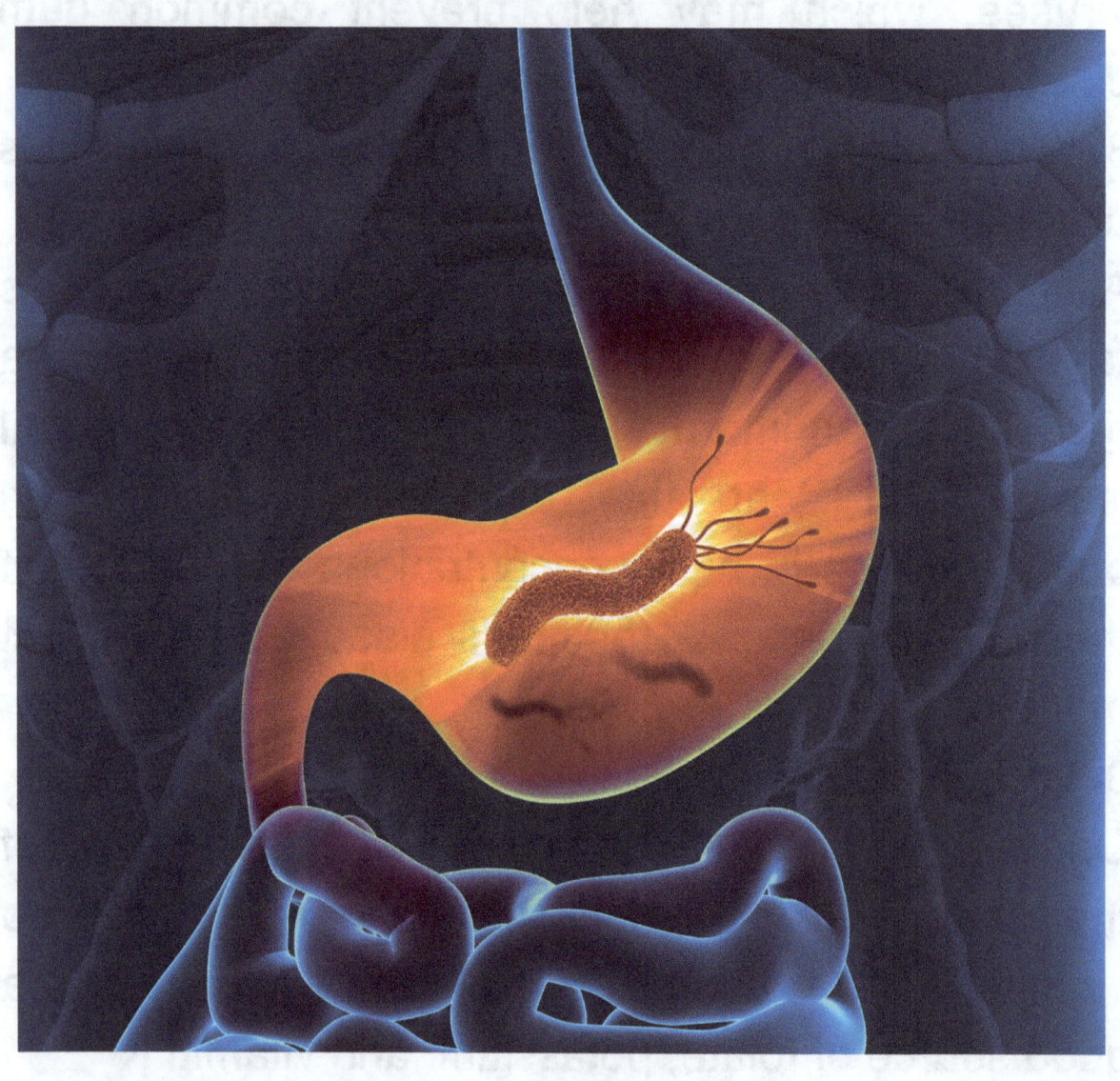

Pomegranate damage to the stomach: do you outweigh its benefits?

Does eating pomegranate or drinking pomegranate juice cause damage to the stomach? Learn about pomegranate damage to the stomach in detail in this article.

Pomegranate damage to the stomach: do you outweigh its benefits?
Pomegranate is one of the most used types of fruits since ancient times due to its many benefits. Continue reading to learn about pomegranate damage to the stomach and the most important information that interests you

Pomegranate damage to the stomach

Eating pomegranate in moderate quantities is safe and does not cause any harm, but in some cases, eating pomegranate or pomegranate juice in large quantities may cause damage to the stomach, including:

1- Irritation of the digestive system.

2- Indigestion.

3- Stomach pain.

4- Bouts of constipation and diarrhea.

5- Vomiting and nausea.

6- Irritation of the lining of the stomach.

Eating pomegranate also causes a number of damages to the body, in addition to pomegranate damage to the stomach, including:

Low blood pressure: Excessive pomegranate consumption causes a drop in blood pressure, especially in people who suffer from blood pressure problems or people who are about to undergo surgery

Food poisoning: Pomegranate peels and stems contain toxic substances, and the use of these parts leads to an attack of food poisoning.

Pharmacological interaction with some medications: Pomegranate intake by some people who take blood-thinning medications or medications to lower blood pressure affects the efficiency of the liver to break down these medications.

Allergic reaction: Some may suffer from pomegranate allergy, and an allergic reaction appears in the form of digestive disorders that include stomach pain and irritation of the stomach lining, itching and swelling, runny nose, and shortness of breath.

benefits of pomegranate

After learning about the damages of pomegranates to the stomach and other damages, let us touch on the benefits of pomegranates and pomegranate juice that outweigh the damages, due to the high nutritional value of pomegranates. Among these benefits are the following

1. Promote heart health

Eating pomegranate contributes to lowering cholesterol levels and preventing its accumulation in the arteries, which accelerates blood flow and prevents hardening and blockage of blood vessels.

2. Strengthening the immune system

The pomegranate content of antioxidants, minerals and vitamins helps fight pathogens and free radicals and prevent cancer, as there are a number of studies confirming the effectiveness of pomegranate in fighting prostate cancer.

3. Memory booster

The antioxidant content of pomegranate contributes to strengthening brain cells, which protects memory and reduces the chance of developing Alzheimer's.

4. Improve digestive health

It was found that pomegranate is beneficial for patients with Crohn's disease and irritable bowel syndrome, as it reduces inflammation and irritation of the intestines

5. Preventing arthritis

There are compounds in pomegranate that prevent joint inflammation and cartilage damage.

6. It inhibits the growth of microbes

Because pomegranate has a group of nutrients, such as: vitamin C and vitamin E, which fight the growth and reproduction of viruses and bacteria.

7. Regulate blood sugar level

Pomegranate contributes to reducing insulin resistance, and this contributes to lowering blood sugar levels

Tips to take advantage of the benefits of pomegranate and avoid its harm

It is possible to benefit from the health benefits of pomegranate and avoid its harm by eating pomegranate in appropriate quantities and following a set of tips, including:

Avoid exposing the pomegranate to heat by heating, as the pomegranate fruit loses part of the nutritional value.

Choose ripe pomegranates that have a heavy size and firm skin.

Eat pomegranate by adding the seeds to salads, yogurt, oatmeal, or desserts.

Prepare fresh pomegranate juice at home, because ready-made juice contains high amounts of sugar and sodium.

Scatter pomegranate seeds on baking paper and freeze them for two hours, then put them in nylon bags for freezing when storing pomegranate seeds, as this method guarantees a long shelf life for pomegranate seeds that may reach a year

Benefits of drinking pomegranate molasses on an empty stomach

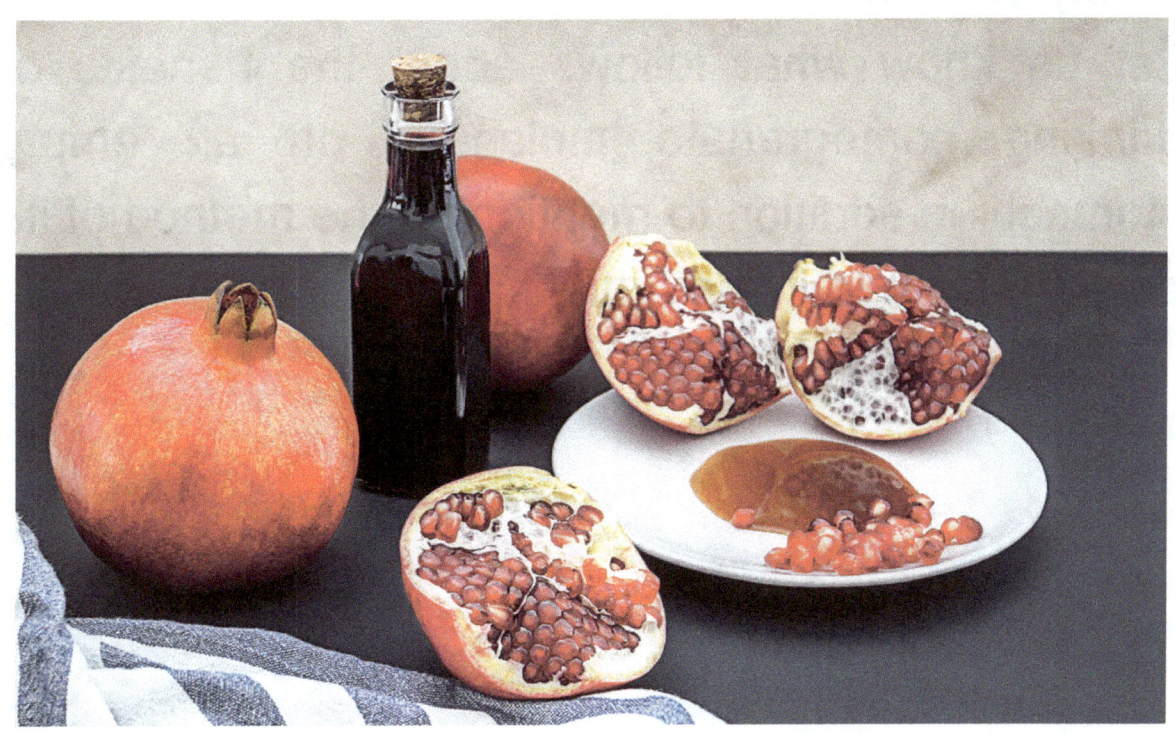

Benefits of drinking pomegranate molasses on an empty stomach

Do you want to know the benefits of drinking pomegranate molasses on an empty stomach? Then you just have to read the article, it will explain all the benefits in addition to teaching you the home preparation method of this molasses.

Benefits of drinking pomegranate molasses on an empty stomach
Let us know what follows about the benefits of drinking pomegranate molasses on an empty stomach, in addition to mentioning the method of its preparation and its potential harm to some

Benefits of drinking pomegranate molasses on an empty stomach

First of all, it should be known that the benefits of drinking pomegranate molasses on an empty stomach are the same as its benefits when drinking it at any time. There is no scientific evidence or research showing that the benefits are different when drinking this molasses on an empty stomach. The most prominent benefits of drinking pomegranate molasses are as follows:

Contribute to reducing the risk of cancer

It was found that pomegranates generally contain high levels of antioxidants equal to 3 times the antioxidants found in green tea, and this is evidence of the ability of pomegranate molasses to contribute to resisting free radicals, the main cause of various types of cancer

Strengthening the body's immunity

Pomegranate provides the body with 40% of your daily vitamin C needs, as well as pomegranate molasses provides vitamin C for the body, but at a lower rate, being exposed to heating, which reduces this percentage, and whatever the ratio is, once the body obtains vitamin C, immunity will be strengthened and increased.

Protection from heart disease

Protecting the heart from diseases when drinking pomegranate molasses came because of its ability to:

1- Increase blood flow in the blood vessels.

2- Slowing the growth of plaques on the walls of the arteries.

3- Reducing cholesterol levels in the blood.

Alzheimer's disease prevention

One of the benefits of drinking pomegranate molasses on an empty stomach or at any other time is that it enhances the health of brain cells, and this makes it resistant to future mental diseases, the most important of which is Alzheimer's

Promote digestive health

Pomegranate, its juice and molasses all provide good health for the digestive system, as they reduce gastritis and improve the digestion process, and all these products are useful for relieving the symptoms of the following diseases:

Crohn's disease.

Ulcerative colitis.

Inflammatory bowel diseases.

Reducing inflammation in the body

Since pomegranate molasses is rich in antioxidants, this may indicate its ability to reduce the severity of some infections in the body, including wound infections and intestinal infections, as mentioned above.

Pomegranate molasses also contributes to relieving arthritis, because it contains flavonols

Reduce weight

The ability of pomegranate molasses to reduce weight is a potential benefit for humans to this day, as the study that was conducted on this molasses concerned mice that were given 4 milliliters of pomegranate molasses for 11 weeks, so that the result was a decrease in their weights. We hope to conduct many studies that concern humans to confirm This benefit or deny it.

Other benefits

You can also get the following benefits of drinking pomegranate molasses on an empty stomach:

Reducing high blood pressure.
Providing many important vitamins for the body.
Increase skin glow

How to prepare pomegranate molasses

To reap the benefits of drinking pomegranate molasses on an empty stomach and at other times, it is preferable to prepare it at home in the following way:

1- Peel the pomegranate seeds and take the resulting ones.

2- Mix the pomegranate seeds with an electric mixer.

3- The resulting juice is filtered and the juice is taken.

4- The juice is put on the fire, and two tablespoons of sugar and a little lemon juice are added to each cup.

5- Reduce the heat to the juice and leave it for one hour.

6- The molasses is removed from the heat and left aside until it cools down, then it is filled in containers.

It is worth noting that every 10 kilos of pomegranate produces approximately one kilo of pomegranate molasses

Pomegranate molasses damage

The damages that will be mentioned in the following for pomegranate molasses are the same as the harms of eating pomegranates, as they both have the same effect on the body:

Exposure to an allergic reaction

Many people are allergic to pomegranate and its products, and as soon as they eat a little of it, they are exposed to one of the forms of allergy, including: rash, itching, shortness of breath, and runny nose.

Interaction with some medications

Pomegranate molasses, as well as pomegranate, have the ability to interact with many medications, including: high blood pressure medications, and medications that are processed inside the liver, so care must be taken when combining drinking pomegranate molasses with taking medications

Introducing high calories to the body

Pomegranate molasses, which is bought ready-made, contains very high levels of sugar when prepared, and this makes it rich in calories that cause weight gain if not consumed.

Digestion problems

It is known that pomegranate molasses is a concentrated ingredient with an acidic taste, so drinking it on an empty stomach can cause a feeling of heartburn, and it can also cause digestion problems. In such cases, it is recommended to drink it at other times to avoid these risks

Benefits of pomegranate molasses for slimming: Get to know them

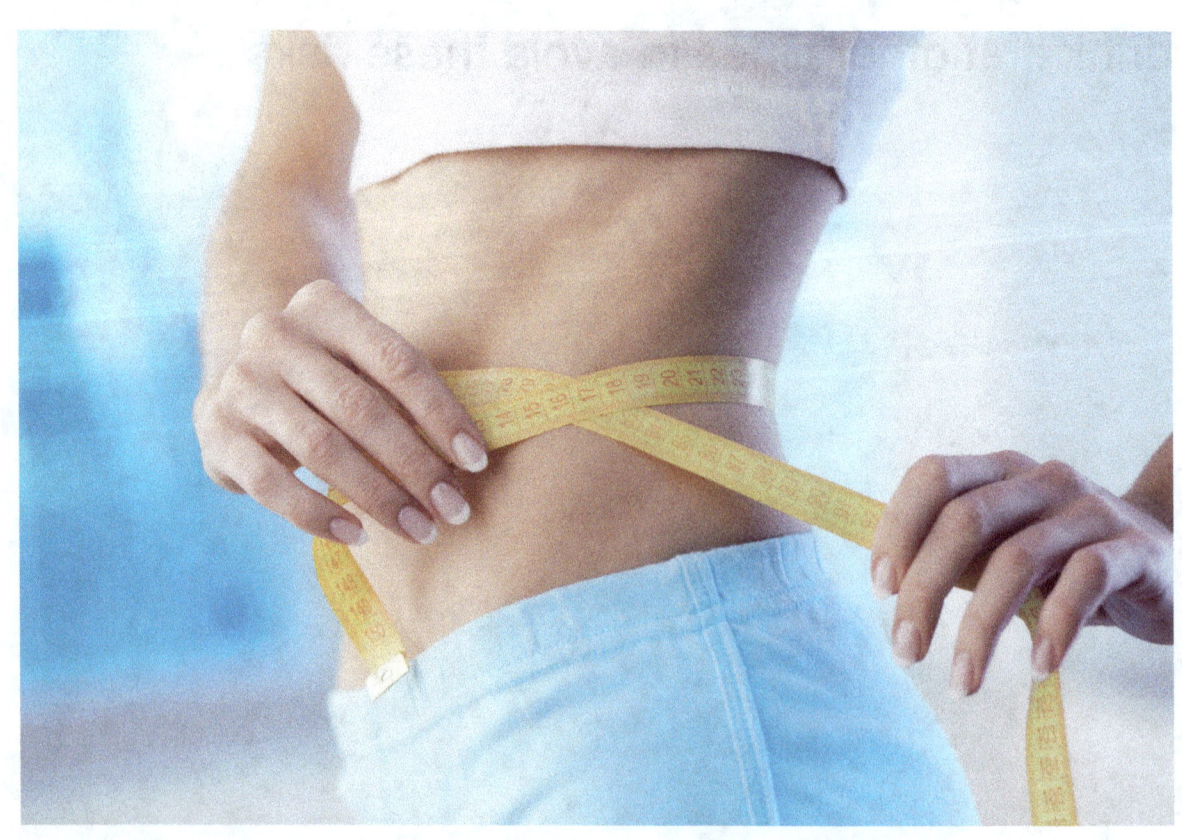

Benefits of pomegranate molasses for slimming: Get to know them

Can pomegranate molasses help in weight loss? In this article, you have the most important information about the benefits of pomegranate molasses for slimming.

Benefits of pomegranate molasses for slimming: Get to know them

Let's learn about the benefits of pomegranate molasses for slimming and other benefits:

Benefits of pomegranate molasses for slimming

A study conducted on mice indicated the role of pomegranate molasses in losing weight, due to the richness of pomegranate molasses in polyphenol compounds, which give it good antioxidant properties compared to fresh pomegranate juice. For example, the study showed that pomegranate molasses contains 252.28 mg eq / liter of acid Gallic acid, while the percentage of the same compound ranged at about 79.49 mg eq / liter in fresh pomegranate juice

So, the antioxidant properties and the ability of pomegranate molasses to fight free radicals, reduce the percentage of triglycerides, and inhibit the process of fat oxidation helped in a clear decrease in weight, but of course, more research is still required to prove the information more and more clearly and to ensure that this is true.

Other benefits of pomegranate molasses
In addition to the benefits of pomegranate molasses for slimming, it has other potential health benefits, including the following:
1. Provides the body with minerals and vitamins
Pomegranate molasses contains a variety of important vitamins and minerals, including: manganese, magnesium, copper, vitamin B6, selenium, potassium, iron, and calcium.
2. It helps to strengthen the blood
Pomegranate molasses may contribute to strengthening the blood, by increasing the number and size of red blood cells, and raising the level of hemoglobin, thus helping to relieve symptoms of anemia and its complications

182

3. Promotes healthy skin

The antioxidant properties of pomegranate molasses help protect the skin from premature sagging and wrinkles, and the presence of vitamin B3 in pomegranate molasses contributes to maintaining the elasticity and freshness of the skin.

4. It gives health to the hair

The permanent use of pomegranate molasses provides the body with minerals that are important for the health and strength of hair. It contributes to stimulating the growth of hair follicles and leads to adding shine and health to the appearance of hair in general.

5. Relieves digestive disorders

Containing vitamin B in pomegranate molasses helps regulate the functioning of the digestive nervous system, thus improving bowel movement, regulating digestion, and reducing constipation, bloating, abdominal pain, and spasms

6. Promotes a healthy immune system
Pomegranate molasses may affect the production of white blood cells and stimulate their production, which contributes to strengthening the immune system and fighting infections and various microbes.

7. It improves bone health
The fact that pomegranate molasses contains iron, copper, and selenium works to strengthen bones and improve their health, and its containment of calcium helps in bone growth and protection from fragility.

8. Promotes heart health
Pomegranate molasses affects heart health by helping to lower high blood pressure because it contains potassium, and by reducing harmful cholesterol and raising the level of beneficial cholesterol in the blood, thus preventing atherosclerosis and its complications

How to make homemade pomegranate molasses
Homemade pomegranate molasses can be made through the following steps:

Mix a liter of pomegranate juice with 1/2 cup of lemon juice and 1/2 cup of sugar.
Put the mixture on the fire and wait for it to boil.
Reduce the heat and keep stirring until the mixture has reduced by half and its color has turned dark.
Leave the pomegranate molasses aside for 45 minutes, then pour it into a glass jar and keep it in the fridge.
Pomegranate molasses damage
After we explained the benefits of pomegranate molasses for slimming and other health problems, and despite the degree of safety of eating it, the alert about some warnings is important, including the following

1. High blood sugar

Although pomegranate molasses is a good alternative to processed sugars for diabetics, excessive consumption of it may negatively affect their sugar level.

2. Diarrhea

Excessive consumption of pomegranate molasses may also lead to diarrhea and worsening of pomzoe symptoms

Pomegranate molasses damage: do you outweigh its benefits?

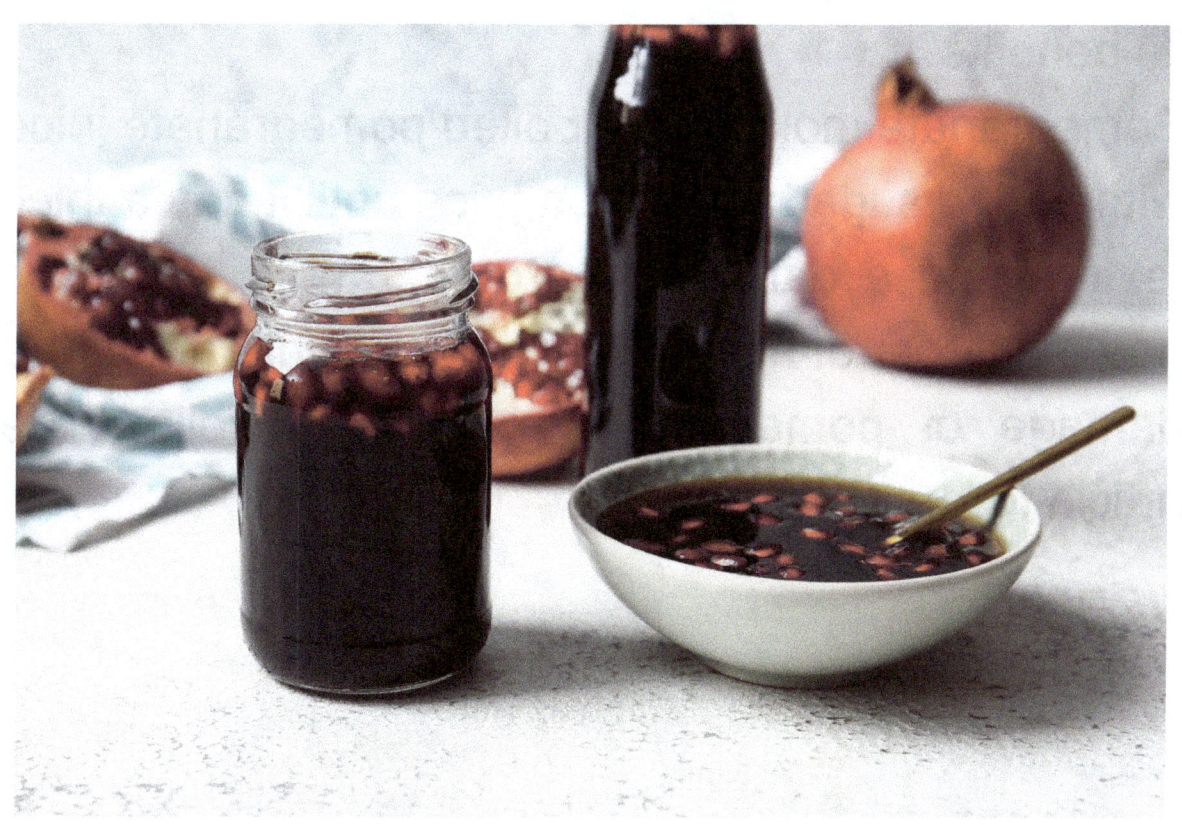

Pomegranate molasses damage: do you outweigh its benefits?

Recently, the use of natural sweeteners instead of artificial ones such as pomegranate molasses has increased, but what are the harms of pomegranate molasses? Are there benefits to using it? Here is the answer in the following article.

Pomegranate molasses damage: do you outweigh its benefits?

Pomegranate molasses is boiled pomegranate juice with added sugar and lemon juice until it has a thick texture and a dark color. Pomegranate molasses has a number of health benefits, but what about the damage of pomegranate molasses? Follow the article to know the answer

Pomegranate molasses damage

There are no scientific studies at the present time that prove the existence of pomegranate molasses damage, but there are a set of precautions that must be adhered to when eating pomegranate molasses as a kind of intense sweetener, to avoid any damage resulting from the use of pomegranate or intense sweeteners in general, despite its safe use in quantities Moderate.

As it is likely that there will be a group of pomegranate molasses damages associated with the side effects of pomegranate or intense sweeteners in general, and these damages are explained as follows:

1. Pomegranate damage

Side effects of using pomegranate:

an allergic reaction

Some may suffer from an allergy to pomegranate, which leads to an allergic reaction represented by difficulty breathing, itching, swelling and runny nose, so it is advised to avoid pomegranate extracts by this group

food poisoning

The roots, stems, and peels of pomegranate fruits contain toxic substances, so you should avoid eating or squeezing them together with pomegranate seeds when making molasses.

Reduction of Blood pressure

The use of pomegranate and its extracts causes a drop in blood pressure, especially in people who suffer from low blood pressure problems, and eating it before any surgery may cause a loss of control of blood pressure, which leads to surgical problems, so it is advised to avoid taking any of the pomegranate extracts before Two weeks from the date of the operation.

drug interaction

In case of using any of the medications to control cholesterol levels or regulate blood pressure, you should avoid using pomegranate extracts because it causes inhibition of the speed and work of the liver to break down these medications

2. The damage of pomegranate molasses as an intense sweetener

Although sweeteners are an excellent alternative to using refined sugars, there are some damages that may result from excessive use, which may cause damage to pomegranate molasses. These damages are explained as follows:

High sugar levels: Excessive use of pomegranate molasses as an intense sweetener causes high blood sugar levels, especially in diabetics.

Severe bouts of diarrhea: Using large amounts of intense sweeteners causes diarrhea and loose stools.

Digestive problems: People who suffer from Irritable Bowel Syndrome (IBS), may suffer from a disorder and discomfort in the digestive system.

Benefits of pomegranate molasses

After discussing the possible harms of pomegranate molasses, let us learn about the potential benefits of pomegranate molasses, as follows

Strengthening immunity

Because pomegranate molasses is rich in antioxidants and vitamin C, this boosts the production of white blood cells, which are the first line of defense of the immune system.

Reducing cholesterol levels

The polyphenols found in pomegranate molasses reduce the level of harmful cholesterol in the body, and this reduces the chance of atherosclerosis, strokes and heart attacks.

Improve the health of various body systems

Pomegranate molasses stock is high in vitamin B, and this improves the health of the muscular, nervous and digestive systems, and contributes to the promotion of normal growth and development.

Increase skin glasses

The content of pomegranate molasses in vitamin C and antioxidants contributes to improving skin health and reducing oxidative stress that causes premature signs of aging such as aging and wrinkles

Strengthening hair follicles

Pomegranate molasses contains a group of minerals and organic substances that improve hair health by enhancing the durability of hair follicles and increasing the luster of hair locks.

Prepare pomegranate molasses at home to avoid its damage

It is possible to prepare pomegranate molasses at home, following the following method:

the components

We need the following ingredients:

1 liter of pomegranate juice.
1/2 cup of lemon juice.
1/2 cup of sugar

How to prepare

Follow these steps to prepare pomegranate molasses at home:

1- Mix the three ingredients together well, and leave the mixture on the gas until it boils.

2- Allow the mixture to boil until it becomes homogeneous and reaches the desired density.

3- Stir the mixture until it becomes dark in color.

4- Leave the mixture to cool for 45 minutes.

5- Pour the mixture into a tightly closed glass container.

6- Keep pomegranate molasses in the refrigerator, preferably within 6 months

Pomegranate vinegar: Here are the benefits and method of preparation

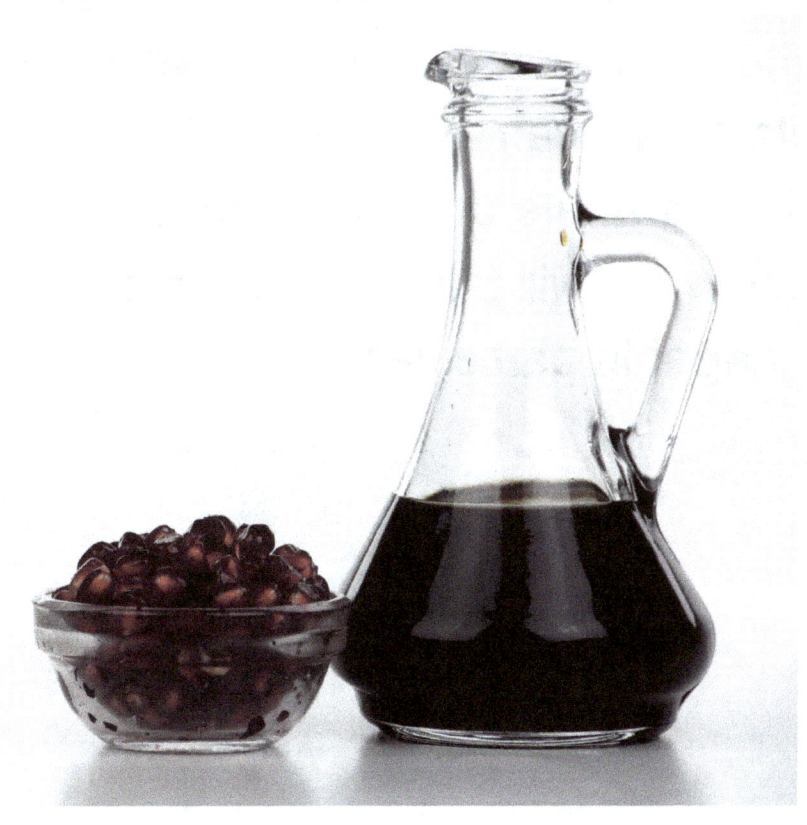

Pomegranate vinegar: Here are the benefits and method of preparation

In this article, we will learn about the benefits of pomegranate vinegar, its uses, and how to prepare it at home, along with its side effects.

Pomegranate vinegar: Here are the benefits and method of preparation
Pomegranate contains a high percentage of vitamins, potassium and antioxidants, and these elements can be obtained either by eating fresh pomegranate or in the form of juice or vinegar, and below we will talk in more detail about pomegranate vinegar in particular

Benefits of pomegranate vinegar

Vinegar prepared from pomegranate may provide the following benefits:

1. Helps lower blood cholesterol

This vinegar can help prevent the accumulation of cholesterol in the arteries thanks to its richness in antioxidants, especially polyphenols, tannins, anthocyanins, and ellagic acid, which have a positive effect in reducing low-density lipoprotein and improving Heart health.

2. Contributes to lowering blood pressure

Since it may prevent hardening of the arteries, it may also affect systolic blood pressure levels, and this benefit may be attributed to the tannins and antioxidants that provide the necessary protection for the heart and blood vessels.

Potassium is believed to have a role in lowering blood pressure and improving blood flow as well

3. Enhance memory and mood

This vinegar contains a percentage of flavonoids that have an effective role in protecting memory and promoting brain health, as it is a type of antioxidant that contributes to controlling free radicals that cause mood disorders, depression, and memory deterioration, especially in the elderly.

In addition, vinegar contains estrone, a form of estrogen whose effect studies have not yet shown as an alternative treatment for synthetic hormones for women prone to mood swings in menopause.

4. It may play a role in fighting cancer

Vinegar may slow the growth of cancer and can reduce the volume of blood flowing to tumors.

5. Enhancing the functioning of the digestive system

Vinegar contains acetic acid, which enhances the absorption of nutrients from the food eaten

6. Improve body health

When the nutrients the body needs, especially minerals, are absorbed, the body will be able to fight cancer, diabetes, and osteoporosis.

7. Helps reduce weight

A study conducted on mice that adopted a high-fat diet proved that consuming pomegranate vinegar may contribute to losing excess weight and fighting obesity.

8. Improve calcium absorption

People who suffer from lactose intolerance need alternative sources of calcium, and eating this vinegar will help absorb calcium when eating foods rich in it

How to make pomegranate vinegar

To prepare vinegar at home instead of buying it ready-made, you can follow the following steps:

1- Sterilize a jar in boiling water for 15 minutes, then let it dry.

2- Put 2 cups of white vinegar on the stove and leave it until it gets hot only without boiling.

3- Put 1 cup of pomegranate seeds in a jar, cover it with warm vinegar, cover it tightly and leave it in the sunlight for about 8-10 days, then store it in a cool and dark place for up to 3 months.

pomegranate vinegar uses

There are several ways in which vinegar prepared from pomegranate can be used, including:

Dipping Sauce: Add it to olive oil and use as a dip.

Drink: Add 1-2 tablespoons of pomegranate vinegar to 1 cup of water, and drink it in the morning, before bed, or during meals

Pickling: Substitute regular vinegar for pomegranate vinegar for pickling vegetables.

Salad Dressing: Try adding vinegar on its own to a salad, or mix it with olive oil, garlic, or mustard for a flavor boost.

Cooking: Season soups, chicken, meat, and fish with vinegar.

Pomegranate vinegar damage

Since this vinegar is made from pomegranates, its damages are the same as the damages caused by pomegranates, whether when ingested or applied to the skin, and are summarized as follows:

1- Itching.
2- Swelling.
3- Difficulty breathing.
4- Runny nose

Prepare and compose
Professor / Radwan Abu Bakr
All copyrights reserved to the author .© 2023

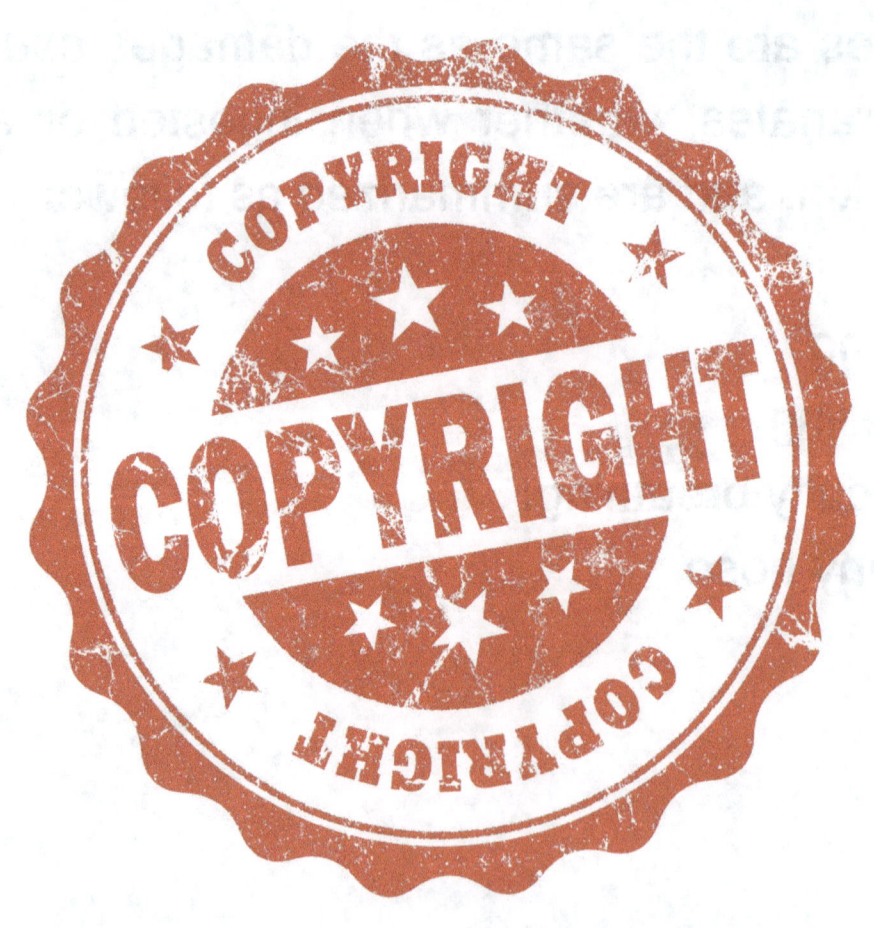

www.ingramcontent.com/pod-product-compliance
Lightning Source LLC
Chambersburg PA
CBHW080827220526
45467CB00008B/2218